SOUTHERN
FOLK
MEDICINE

SOUTHERN
FOLK
MEDICINE

HEALING TRADITIONS FROM THE
APPALACHIAN FIELDS AND FORESTS

PHYLLIS D. LIGHT
FOREWORD BY ROSEMARY GLADSTAR

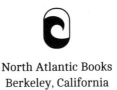

North Atlantic Books
Berkeley, California

Published by   Cover design by Bill Zindel
North Atlantic Books   Interior design by Happenstance Type-O-Rama
Berkeley, California   Printed in the United States of America

Southern Folk Medicine: Healing Traditions from the Appalachian Fields and Forests is sponsored and published by the Society for the Study of Native Arts and Sciences (dba North Atlantic Books), an educational nonprofit based in Berkeley, California, that collaborates with partners to develop cross-cultural perspectives, nurture holistic views of art, science, the humanities, and healing, and seed personal and global transformation by publishing work on the relationship of body, spirit, and nature.

North Atlantic Books' publications are available through most bookstores. For further information, visit our website at www.northatlanticbooks.com or call 800-733-3000.

MEDICAL DISCLAIMER: The following information is intended for general information purposes only. Individuals should always see their health care provider before administering any suggestions made in this book. Any application of the material set forth in the following pages is at the reader's discretion and is his or her sole responsibility.

Library of Congress Cataloging-in-Publication Data

Names: : Light, Phyllis D., author.
Title: Southern folk medicine : healing traditions from the Appalachian
   fields and forests / Phyllis D. Light.
Description: Berkeley, California : North Atlantic Books, 2018. | Includes
   index.
Identifiers: LCCN 2017039532 (print) | LCCN 2017050448 (ebook) | ISBN
   9781623171575 (e-book) | ISBN 9781623171568 (paperback)
Subjects: LCSH: Traditional medicine—Appalachian Region, Southern. |
   Holistic medicine—Appalachian Region, Southern. | Alternative
   medicine—Appalachian Region, Southern. | Healing—Appalachian Region,
   Southern. | Human geography—Appalachian Region, Southern. |
   Folklore—Appalachian Region, Southern. | BISAC: HEALTH & FITNESS /
   Alternative Therapies. | BODY, MIND & SPIRIT / Healing / General. |
   MEDICAL / Holistic Medicine.
Classification: LCC GR880 (ebook) | LCC GR880 .L53 2018 (print) | DDC
   398.20975—dc23
LC record available at https://lccn.loc.gov/2017039532

3 4 5 6 7 8 9 10 KPC 24 23 22 21 20

This book includes recycled material and material from well-managed forests. North Atlantic Books is committed to the protection of our environment. We print on recycled paper whenever possible and partner with printers who strive to use environmentally responsible practices.

To all my children, Jeremy Griggs,
Jessica Griggs, Ian Harrison, Alan Harrison,
and Raven Light-Priest. And to all my
grandchildren, the ones on the Earth now,
and the ones yet to be. I love you all.

❧ ACKNOWLEDGMENTS ❧

I WOULD LIKE to thank my dear friend Matthew Wood, a wise and talented herbalist who has supported my journey into the vast world of modern herbalism and who always has a willing ear for my latest ah-has about life, herbalism, and the nature of things. I'd like to thank the folks at *Plant Healer Magazine*, Jesse Wolf Hardin and Kiva Rose Bell-Hardin, for their continual love and support and willingness to let me use excerpts from previously published magazine articles in the book. I'd also like to thank David Winston, Madelon Hope, Lesley Shore, Rosemary Gladstar, Karyn Sanders, Bonnie Kreckow, Michael Tierra, Kathleen Maier, and Matthew Briese for all the years of support and belief. I would also like to thank all my students who have urged me to codify this system and save it for the future. A big hug to you all.

❦ CONTENTS ❧

ꕭ FOREWORD ꕭ

WHEN I FIRST met Phyllis Light several years ago at an herb conference, I was fully captivated by this vibrant, enthusiastic herbalist from the South. She was not only brilliant, but also funny, one of the best story tellers ever, and she was completely impassioned, like me, by the plants. We stayed in touch. When Phyllis would phone, I'd make sure there was a enough time for the call. If the weather was nice, I'd take my cup of tea and sit on the porch knowing I was in for a long, satisfying, and always insightful conversation—mostly about plants and healing—but also lavishly sprinkled with details of life, love, and family. In the rural south, for some reason, time doesn't seem as frenzied as elsewhere in the country and Phyllis—the mother of five children and the director of a busy herb school as well as a thriving community herbal practice—always seemed to have enough time for friends, family, and a walk in the woods. I knew I had a lot to learn from this wise woman, not only about plants, but also about life in general.

Following in her father's footsteps and a family lineage that stretched back generations, Phyllis was a "plant person," a healer, and had been studying and practicing herbalism in her hometown in rural Alambama for years before I met her. She had been close friends and an early student of Tommie Bass, a legendary and beloved folk healer. Phyllis, however, had taken what she learned from her teacher one giant step further. As she writes, "Having a culturally diverse clientele helped me to realize that the basic practices of folk medicine are similar regardless of the country of origin, and that in many countries, cross-pollination with other traditions started hundreds if not thousands of years ago." Not only is she carrying on the traditions of folk medicine as it was being practiced in the rural south, she's also integrating it with other traditional folk medicine practices and, perhaps even more significantly, integrating it with modern medical and herbal practices.

When I first invited Phyllis to teach at the prestigious International Herb Symposium at Wheaton College several years ago, she promptly asked to present on Southern folk traditions. At that time outside of the rural south, no one was talking much about Southern Folk Medicine. Instead, most herbalists were intent on "legitimizing" herbalism by emphasizing the scientific research and modern applications of plant medicine. But Phyllis's classes filled up quickly and got excellent reviews. In her well-informed manner and crystal clear voice, she shed new light on an old subject, stimulating interest and bringing credibility to one of our oldest folk traditions, a folk system born and bred in the Deep South.

Until recently, folk medicine and traditional practices—*especially* folk medicine from rural Appalachia—were considered antiquated, outdated, and something only those too poor to obtain modern medicines would ever consider using. Even among the herbal community who generally valued traditional approaches, little credence or attention was given to our Southern Folk Medicine. While both Traditional Chinese Medicine (TCM) and Ayurveda herbalism (India) were diligently studied, and our Western Eclectic medical traditions of the eighteenth and nineteenth centuries were integrated readily into our modern herbal practices, very little thought was given to folk traditions, and Southern Folk Medicine especially was largely ignored by everyone outside of the south. Phyllis was one of a small group of people advocating for Southern Folk Medicine as a legitimate system of healing worthy of attention. As she states, "You don't have to be Southern to learn and use Southern Folk Medicine, any more than you have to be Asian to study and use Traditional Chinese Medicine."

In a world where disease has become so rampart, even in developed countries with presumably more advanced medical techniques, integrating folk traditions that have proven effective over decades of use and are often inexpensive and readily available can bring value to healthcare within communities. Phyllis became a strong voice for these traditional practices through her classes, published articles, and within her clinical practice. Through her persistence, and the work of others like her, Southern Folk Medicine "has found a niche within mainstream medicine in the protocols, techniques, and philosophies of integrative medicine."

Phyllis's fabulous book, *Southern Folk Medicine,* takes another huge step in ensuring that the our healing folk traditions continue to thrive. In this book,

Phyllis does more than just codify and document Southern Folk Medicine. While describing the rich complexity that comprise these traditions, she also presents practical ways to incorporate the best that folk medicine has to offer into our daily health practices. And she presents an integrated approach to healthcare throughout the book advising that no one system stands alone, but that "knowledge should flow across the two domains of science and tradition in a more even, two-way transmission that does not rely on indoctrination in training but rather on observable outcomes in those who are sick."

Southern Folk Medicine, like all traditional healing arts, isn't a static system of health care, but is an ever-changing and evolving body of knowledge. Influenced by the influx of many nationalities through centuries of migration and settlement, it evolved into an integrative and practical system of heathcare, richly textured with a variety of cultural and spiritual beliefs. And that cross-pollination of cultural healing skills continues on through time. Like busy bees flitting from flower to flower, we have the responsibility to integrate the best that these systems have to offer into our modern healthcare and to "pay this information forward." Treasures like *Southern Folk Medicine* will ensure that the richness of this system, *our* very own U.S. tradition born and bred on the turf of the southern states, will continue to have an important place not only in the rural south, but throughout the rich tapestry of modern healthcare systems. On every page, there's a richly told story, a brilliant passage, a bit of wisdom or practical advice about health and healing that make the kind of sense that only folk traditions do. I know I'll be referring to it time and again, and will be incorporating many of her suggestions into my healing practice.

—*Rosemary Gladstar*
Herbalist and Author

❧ PREFACE ❧

IT'S NOT MY Granny's world anymore, nor any other old-time healer's. The whole landscape of medicine has changed in the intervening time since they were young. Herbalists like Tommie Bass didn't see people on multiple medications because no one was taking multiple medications in those days. Today, folks might be on six or more medications at once; back then it was rare for a person to be on any medication for any length of time other than an antibiotic, and multiple medications were considered only for the seriously ill who were close to death. It was the pre-pharmaceutical, pre-medical insurance, pre-vaccination era, at least in this part of the country. Obesity was rare and considered a glandular problem. Folks didn't have very much to eat, especially the amount of food required to become obese, and most everyone had to work at some sort of physical labor to make a living. A person considered a few pounds overweight in those days wouldn't even be noticed in today's population. Access to food was generally limited to what was raised in the garden or farm or hunted in the woods, with a few commodities such as coffee, sugar, flour, and cornmeal bought at the grocery store.

The most common disorders were digestive problems, worms, heart problems, arthritis, women's reproductive issues, the occasional case of high blood sugar, and sinus infections and related issues. Cases of cancer in the community were fairly uncommon and generally diagnosed in the later stages. I remember when a young mother was diagnosed with breast cancer and the whole community was shocked—it was that rare. Cancer was considered an old person's disease, and it was always shocking when a younger person was diagnosed, especially children with leukemia.

But it's a different world now: 68.8 percent of the population of the United States is considered overweight or obese. According to the National Institute of Environmental Health Sciences, it's estimated that about 23.5 million Americans have been diagnosed with an autoimmune disease, but other organizations believes it's closer to fifty million. About 25 percent of the population of the United States is considered too disabled to work. Heart disease kills around 375,000 Americans each year and is the number one killer in the world. Alzheimer's, which was extremely rare in previous times, is now the sixth-leading cause of death in the United States, and it's estimated that between five million and sixteen million Americans have the disease.

All diseases and disorders are on the rise and I don't believe this has anything to do with better diagnostic techniques. The bottom line is that folks just aren't as healthy as they used to be. What's going on? Why aren't we as healthy as our grandparents? The possible influences on the demise of our health as a nation are too many to list and it isn't within the scope of this material to discuss this broad topic. But something has to change, something has to shift; we can't go on like this.

I've no doubt that traditional knowledge, such as herbalism, has a place in this shift. We need every single modality in our knowledge base to improve the health of our country and the world. Somehow, folk traditions and science must find a meeting ground.

Where is the place that science and traditional knowledge can come together in the best interests of our health? In broad terms, science refers to the body of knowledge about the phenomena of the natural world. In modern terms, science also refers to a system of acquiring knowledge based on the scientific method, to the organized body of knowledge gained by such research, and to a particular field or domain of systematic inquiry in which such knowledge is sought. For many people, the belief in science is the basis of all healthcare, though folks are beginning to understand its limitations.

There is also traditional knowledge that has been used for centuries as part of the healthcare system. I do like anthropologist Martha Johnson's definition of Traditional Ecological Knowledge (TEK), which includes the category of folk medicine: "a body of knowledge built by a group of people through generations living in close contact with nature. It includes a system of classification, a set of empirical observations about the local environment, and a system of self-management that governs resource use."

Folk traditions have thousands of years of empirical evidence to validate methods and use. Though traditional knowledge is not formed through the scientific method, it may contain common elements such as observation. It is based on the collective experience of generations as well as the immediate experience of the practitioner. There is usually no real separation between secular and sacred knowledge.

Traditional medicines, such as Southern Folk Medicine, are not static, but are evolving and changing through synthesis and hybridization to meet the needs of its people, the communities or groups that still practice some aspect of traditional medicines. For example, Native Americans quickly learned to use the plants brought from Europe by the settlers once these plants escaped from gardens into the wild. Some Native American groups believed that European diseases could only be cured by using the plants from the land in which the disease originated. For this reason, they turned to European plants to treat diseases of European origin that they contracted from the settlers.

It is very difficult to codify a body of knowledge, such as Southern Folk Medicine, without losing some of its original characteristics. As an oral tradition, some information is lost with each new generation, but at the same time, new information becomes available as the needs of the people change, new populations move into the system, or the system moves into other cultures. You don't have to be Southern to learn and use Southern Folk Medicine, any more than you have to be Asian to study and use Traditional Chinese Medicine.

With today's disorders and diseases, I believe an integrated approach offers the best healthcare for the citizens of this country and of the world. No one wants to live without modern medicine and what it has to offer. Think of how many lives are saved each year from the use of antibiotics! But there is also benefit to be found in herbalism, nutrition, and the use of home remedies that is being ignored. To be the most effective, knowledge should flow across the two domains of science and tradition in a more even, two-way transmission that does not rely on indoctrination in training but rather on observable outcomes in those who are sick. Isn't that what really matters? Shouldn't people who are sick feel better, have less pain, and attain a better quality of life? Shouldn't that be the bottom line?

Let's not throw out the baby with the bath water. It's going to take a lot of work to get this country and the world in a healthy place. We need all the resources and all the help we can get.

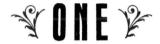

ONE

What Is Folk Medicine?

I'm just trying to give some ease.
—*Tommie Bass, nationally acclaimed*
folk herbalist from Sand Rock, Alabama

WE PARKED THE truck on top of Billy Ridge at the crack of dawn to go ginseng hunting down the mountainside. The early cool of the September air was crisp and clean as we zigzagged our way down the mountain, cutting a path through the understory brush and along the ravines. Granddaddy Light carried a walking stick cut from a young sapling to ease his old bones through the woods and to fend off snakes. His hands shook with palsy and his steps were slow, so we moved at a leisurely pace to accommodate his affliction. Daddy carried the ginseng or sang hoe over his right shoulder and a burlap sack in the other hand. The sang hoe had a pick on one side and a half a hoe blade on the other and could be used to dig deep into the dirt and lift out a root.

As the day wore on, we had nothing to show for all our morning's effort. No sang had been found. *Sang* is short for American ginseng and is a term which is used throughout Appalachia. Everyone was feeling a bit glum and a bit tired as we rested on the big rocks around the blue hole outside a Cotaco Valley cave, grateful for the deep shade of the densely packed trees around the sinkhole. Tangled fishing line littered the lower branches, signs of failed attempts to cast for the fish that swam between the blue hole outside the cave and its sister blue hole inside.

Caving was one of my favorite activities, having been introduced at a young age by my father. This particular cave was alluring—its great room was magnificent, with a cathedral ceiling that seemed to stretch upward forever. On the far cave wall, intricate rock formations created a water fountain effect with little pools of water flowing from one smaller pool at the top of the cave wall downward to the next larger pool, and on until it reached the largest pool at the cave's floor. In the middle of the great groom was the blue hole, a sinkhole filled with fresh water. No one knew how deep it was, only that it connected to a similar one outside the cave.

But today, there was no time for caving; ginseng was an important source of cash income and the day was getting on. Empty-handed, we headed back toward the truck, a long walk up the north face of the mountain on an overgrown and long-deserted roadbed. Little shrubby pine trees and greenbrier poked up here and there on the old roadbed, the forest reclaiming its land. Down one side of the road was a deep wash, formed by many years of rain rushing down the mountain. This old road had never been paved, having only been used by the folks who had once lived in the settlement at the mountain's plateau shelf.

As we headed back up, I spotted a solitary chimney in the woods and went over to investigate. The chimney (or chimley, in local terms) was all that was left standing from a house in a once prosperous settlement. The houses had been abandoned years ago when a new road was built a few miles to the east, bypassing the lowest part of the valley which was prone to flooding. The owner of the general store had abandoned the settlement, resettling on the new road. The people had followed the store, packing up and moving, abandoning their wooden shacks and chicken coops to the workings of nature. For you see, the people had never owned the land their houses were on. The vast acreage was all owned by one family, as was the general store. They rented to tenant farmers who worked the cotton fields in the valley below. Soon only stone chimneys and fallen-down buildings stood as reminders that people had once occupied the land and that cotton was no longer king.

Abandoned homesteads were always an exciting discovery, and exploring them was one of my favorite activities. To explore the sites where people had once lived, raised their children, and buried their dead was the most intriguing activity in the world. Sometimes, the houses were abandoned, with all the furniture and house goods left inside. This happened when elderly parents died and their children, now living in other states, had no time to rescue possessions left behind in the backwoods of Alabama. These old houses and their belongings could sit for years and years until the land was finally sold and new owners took possession.

My brother Norman and I loved to do this type of exploring. Once, in similar circumstances, we had found an old trunk full of women's clothes from the early 1900s. What an amazing treasure! You just never knew what you might find in abandoned houses. On this day, I found an old fruit jar, discovered several small bottles which had once held patent medicines and hair tonic, and unearthed a handful of marbles. To a child, these were amazing discoveries which I would later flaunt to younger siblings and cousins.

There were usually fruit and nut trees around the old settlements and homesteads, and this was no exception. The pear tree was ripe with fruit already falling thick on the ground, and a muscadine (wild grape) vine clung to the last of its thick-skinned yield not yet eaten by the birds or possums. Both would make wonderful jellies, preserves, and syrups. Abandoned settlements were also good places to find herbs, especially in the cleared areas around old chicken coops or pig pens.

I was so intent on my explorations that I jumped when Daddy shouted for me to "Come on!" They had found some sang.

Every plant has an ally, a companion, and a use. As we dug the ginseng, Granddaddy said that ginseng, deer, and rattlesnakes are often found together. Granddaddy talked really, really slow, partially because of his palsy and partially just because that was the way he talked. Any story that Granddaddy started could take awhile. He talked slower than molasses running uphill on a snowy day, as the old saying goes. Sometimes his pauses would be so long that you'd think he had finished the story and so you would start talking. Then Granddaddy would suddenly get his wind back and, with great indignation for being interrupted, finish his story. It was disconcerting, but taught us patience and gave us all good listening skills.

According to Granddaddy, deer eat the ginseng seeds and the seeds pass on through and drop as the deer move around the woods. The seeds then roll down the sides of the mountain until they rest on land that is level enough and moist enough for them to grow. And that's one way ginseng travels around the woods to new locations. That's why following deer trails often leads to ginseng.

Rattlesnakes make winter nests in the sides of mountains near ginseng patches but above wet ground, and they are looking for their winter's nests about the same time ginseng is ready to dig. Most ginseng hunters run up on at least one or two rattlesnakes during a season. According to legend, because rattlesnakes and ginseng live so close together and share the same land, they made a pact. If you injure one, the other extracts revenge; what you do to one, you do to the other. Killing a rattlesnake is always bad luck; the spirits don't like that. And even worse, if you harm a snake, the ginseng can stop working for you.

We finished gathering the sang and were almost back at the truck when we heard the rattle. It was a granddaddy rattlesnake coiled right in the middle of the old roadbed and ready to strike. Daddy moved to one side of the snake and Granddaddy walked over and stood between it and me.

"Shoo, old snake, we don't want no trouble," Granddaddy said. But the snake stayed coiled, rattling its tail.

"It's too late for talking," Daddy said, "it's done hissed at me." Daddy picked up a big rock, ready to deal with that rattlesnake.

"Get to the truck," Daddy said, motioning me onward. But I was frozen, staring at the evil-looking, arrowhead-shaped snake head. "Go on," I said. And I knew he meant it this time and so I headed toward the truck, giving the snake a wide berth. With one last look back, I saw Daddy draw back his throwing arm and I knew we had seen the last of that old snake. Daddy had a fearless attitude about handling snakes or killing poisonous ones. He had been known to grab a snake by the tail, swing it around and around and pop off its head with a whip-like action. He also liked to keep a rat snake or corn snake in his tool shed to keep down the rats. It also kept Mama out of his shed too. She was extremely afraid of snakes.

With Granddaddy's story fresh in my mind, I knew that killing the rattlesnake was bad luck, and I was worried about what might happen to Daddy if he killed the snake. I called out to him, but he just motioned me toward the truck, his eyes never leaving the snake. They were in a contest and there would be only one winner. And that was the end of that old snake.

Ginseng was the only medicinal plant my Daddy ever used until late in his life when his brother B.J. moved to northern Florida and sent him an aloe vera plant and a gallon of aloe vera juice. After that, Daddy said that aloe vera did what ginseng couldn't do, and he would sit in his easy chair and rub aloe vera on all the spots on his skin. Both Daddy and Granddaddy felt that ginseng, in the right amount, could do most everything. I spent years learning those amounts and those uses.

I ate my first ginseng when I was only a little girl. It was fresh dug from the ground, and the smell of the rich-woods dirt filled my nostrils as I took a bite. I was taught to chew on a tidbit of the woody root…slowly…savoring every drop of its sweet bitterness. I could keep a bit of sang in my mouth for hours, worrying it around and around the way a cow chews a cud.

We always kept some dried ginseng in a kitchen drawer, the one where all the odds and ends of the kitchen end up. There among the matches, can openers, screws, and receipts were the dried broken bits of the sang that were too small to sell. The collection grew every year. I still have a few of those broken sang roots, given to me by Mama when Daddy died of an unusual blood cancer that reminded me of the bite of a rattlesnake. They were a last gift and reminder of those precious times in the woods. The roots are as hard as a rock, and many have been dried thirty years or longer, but I can still chew on one for quite some time, letting the sweet bitterness fill my mouth, conjuring up memories of life the way it used to be.

Living with a plant, the way I did ginseng, is the perfect way to get to know it and for it to know you. Ginseng has its own personality, a quality that permeates its medicine, affecting all levels of the body. It can be wiry and tough, offering armor against invasion, keeping out that which is not needed. At the same time, ginseng can be gentle, influencing the body on a deep, cellular level, supporting the immune system and fortifying the spirit. As with many herbs, the dose makes the difference. As a tonic, a little ginseng each day, just a little, supports the body and improves health.

Producing only two or three seed heads each year, ginseng uses its energy wisely, storing most of its vitality in the roots. Ginseng likes to grow on the north side of the mountains in well-drained soil, but will grow in most any hardwood forests. And unlike other herbs of the woods, ginseng, the King of Herbs, is not merely harvested or gathered, but rather it is hunted. Hunting implies that the plant has an innate intelligence which is used to hide or defend itself from attack and capture. Granny Light told me that ginseng, or Little Man, is smart and can become invisible unless it wants to be gathered. And from my experience, I believe this to be true.

Ginseng is sneaky. You can be standing in the middle of a patch and not even know it. Or sometimes you can walk around and around a patch before you realize it's there. But on rare and glorious occasions, you can just walk into the woods and there it appears at your feet, in total welcome and acceptance. Sang has a rare mysterious and magical quality. When I was young, I was sure that ginseng could just pick up and walk through the rich wood's dirt to evade capture.

Sanging is a magical word itself, being used as both a verb and a noun. That day, we went sanging together, and later Granddaddy would tell the rest of the family about the sang. As you might have gathered, ginseng hunting was an annual event in our family that was anticipated with excitement and enthusiasm.

Every sanger has his or her own way of hunting the plant, a system they felt sure would work. I was taught to look for running water, deer trails, and rattlesnakes as signs or markers that sang was nearby. I also learned that little flat ledges on the sides of the mountains often hold the plant. My gin-seng education included instructions to never take all the plants in a patch but to leave some for future growth. I was also taught to break off and replant the arm of the ginseng plant for immediate growth. This is something that modern ginseng hunters don't do—the international market requires the root to be intact. This has sped the decline of wild ginseng populations because hunters aren't replanting. And I understood the necessity of keeping my ginseng patch secret, because others might steal every single plant if they could find them.

No matter their favorite methods of ginseng hunting, everyone in the family agreed that ginseng is found in the snakiest places. Aunt Jewel was known to wear heavy Army boots with metal stove pipes tied around her lower legs to pro-tect against rattlesnake bites. She would often brag about how many strikes she heard pinging against the metal pipes as she walked through the snaky brush.

My uncle Waylon continued to hunt ginseng after my Daddy had stopped, carrying on until his heart and legs just couldn't make their way up and down the mountain slopes anymore. Waylon was little and dark, with the coloring of a Creek Indian, the face of an Irishman, and the fiery temper of both. He fought for and protected his ginseng patch with knife and wits, and few old hunters wanted to cross him in the woods. When Uncle Waylon was in the hospital, nearing the end of his life, I had the opportunity to hear tales of ginseng hunts from the older men who came to visit him. It was a rough-and-tumble business, and people protected their patches fiercely. Money was scarce and herbs like ginseng, pink root, butterfly weed, button snakeroot, and smilax, or greenbrier, brought in much-needed cash. Men earnestly protected the location of herb patches and gathered the plants in secret.

One of the most important lessons in how to find a patch of ginseng took place in Moon Hollow, so named because the only light at night which could be seen shining through the trees was the light of the moon. Moon Hollow, a thousand acres of uninhabited land, was a favorite of ginseng hunters as well as fox hunters. On this particular day in late June, Daddy and I set off to Moon Hollow right after breakfast. He said, "Sister, you need to learn how sang looks at all times of the year if you are going to hunt it." Mama expected us back home by dinnertime (lunch) when food would be on the table promptly at 11 a.m.

Daddy and I passed an abandoned grist mill; the wheel was missing but the apparatus was still there. We continued to hike deeper into the hollow than I had ever been before. We walked and walked, until Daddy suddenly stopped. He pulled a Zane Grey paperback Western novel out of his back pocket and settled himself on the ground at the foot of a big tree and leaned back against the trunk to read.

"Between that tree," he said, pointing, "and that rock and the creek, there are six or seven ginseng plants. Let me know when you find them, Sister." And he started reading.

I looked around me and every plant looked the same: green and about a foot tall. I couldn't locate the ginseng by looking for their red berries; it was only early summer so I didn't have that sign to guide me. I walked around, back and forth between the creek, tree, and rock, but I couldn't find any ginseng.

"Are you sure there are ginseng plants here?" I asked him. "Yup," was the only answer I got.

I looked some more, walking back and forth. I stopped to examine the leaves on a plant. I still couldn't find any ginseng.

"Hurry up, Sister," he said. "It's almost dinnertime." Time was running out.

Frustration is too mild a word to describe how I felt as the morning wore on. "If you're going to learn about herbs," Daddy said, "this is how you learn."

I was about ready to cry. I just couldn't find any ginseng. I stood there, in the middle of all these green plants, closed my eyes, took a breath, and felt the tension leave my body. I just didn't care anymore if I found any plants, and in not caring, I became calm and quiet.

The woods surrounded me. I kept my eyes closed and let my other senses sharpen. I heard the sounds of the birds in the trees and the wind rustling limbs and leaves. I felt the wind as it flowed over my skin. I felt the sun on my head, hot and constant. I smelled the water from the creek and heard its sound moving over the rocks in the creek bed. I smelled the musk and decay from the deep leaf litter on the ground. I heard Daddy breathing and heard the turning of the page in the book he was reading. I smelled life: the life of the land, rich and thick. And in that moment, I became a part of the land too. I couldn't tell where I began and ended or where the land began and ended.

I opened my eyes and the ginseng plants were just glowing, simply glowing. They were vibrantly green as I pointed to them.

"Here they are," I called to Daddy, pointing them out. He stood up, looked to where I pointed and put the book back into his pocket.

"Let's go eat," he said, and that was all the praise or comment I ever got. But that was his way, the Indian way.

And that was how my path with the plants consciously began.

What Is Folk Medicine?

Folk medicine is only one aspect of folkways within a culture. American sociologist William Graham Sumner described folkways as "usages, manners, customs, mores, and morals" which are practiced unconsciously in every culture. David Hackett Fischer in *Albion's Seed: Four British Folkways in America*, describes folkways as, "the normative structure of values, customs, and meanings that exist in any culture." Folkways are the everyday actions that drive our cultures with society.

Folkways can encompass everything aspect of culture, including patterns of speech; ideas of courtship and marriage; ideas on child rearing; beliefs about the supernatural and religion; customs of dress; attitudes toward food and diet; attitudes and beliefs about health, disease, and medicine; attitudes toward time, money, guns, and most other aspects of life. Southern Folk Medicine is one of the folkways of the Southeast regional culture in the United States.

Does this mean that only Southerners will benefit from Southern Folk Medicine? Absolutely not! Anyone can learn and use Southern Folk Medicine. Its practices and principles cut across regional cultures in the United States, and actually across global cultures. It's easy to learn, intuitive, and conceived in the English language, so its idioms are common for English speakers especially.

However, just to make sure we're on the same page, some definitions are in order to avoid any confusion. This might seem a little boring, but is necessary to make sure there are no misunderstandings. The following definitions are ones that I use and are fairly standard.

Folk medicine is defined as a system of medicinal beliefs, knowledge, and practices associated with a particular culture or ethnic group. Generally, these techniques have not been scientifically tested; there are no animal or double-blind studies. But they have been used for hundreds or thousands of years, accumulating massive amounts of empirical evidence and information that supports their effectiveness and safety. The emphasis of folk medicine is on prevention of disease through healthy lifestyle behaviors. Remedies that support health are nontoxic and are mind, body, and spirit oriented. Folk medicine may be used by itself or in conjunction with conventional medical practices.

Southern Folk Medicine and Southern Appalachian Folk Medicine (SAFM) are umbrella terms for the folk medicine of the Southern United States. Due to migration patterns immediately after the Civil War and again in the 1960s and 1970s, you can find Southern Folk Medicine in most major cities in the United States, in the Midwest, and northward to the Great Lakes areas.

Hoodo is the herbal and spiritual African-American folkway which is found predominantly in the Deep South but which spread northward during the great migration of blacks out of the South. It is a combination of the spiritual practices of Africa and Europe, mostly Ireland, and Native American uses of the herbs of the New World.

Native American Medicine, in the context of this book, pertains to the remnants of the folk practices of the Cherokees, Creeks, Choctaws, Chickasaws, and Seminoles, or the Five Civilized Tribes of the Southern United States, including their use of herbs which have become a part of the Southern folk healing tradition.

According to the World Health Organization, *Traditional Medicine (TM)* is "the sum total of the knowledge, skills, and practices based on the theories, beliefs, and experiences indigenous to different cultures, whether explicable or not, used in the maintenance of health as well as in the prevention, assessment, improvement, or treatment of physical and mental illnesses." The use of Traditional Medicine may or may not be supported by scientific research. Its use is focused on the needs of the individual, not the needs of the group. Traditional healers, herbalists, spiritual healers, and bonesetters are all types of traditional medicine practitioners.

Also per the World Health Organization, *herbal medicine* is "the use of crude plant material such as leaves, flowers, fruit, seed, stems, wood, bark, roots, rhizomes, or other plant parts which may be entire, fragmented, or powdered. It also refers to the long historical use of these plant remedies to support the healing function of the body. Their use is well established and widely acknowledged to be safe and effective, and may be accepted by national authorities."

An *herbalist* is a person who uses plants, foods, and other natural healing techniques to support good health and the body's innate healing processes. Plants used by herbalists have a broad definition and include not only herbaceous plants but also shrubs, trees, mushrooms, lichens, and fruits and vegetables. A commonality among herbalists is their love of the land and plants, and a feeling of a special connection to the Earth. The herbal perspective is holistic, viewing the body as mind, body, and spirit, all rolled into one.

Natural medicines such as herbs shine in the prevention of illness and the reduction of risk factors for illness. The emphasis is on prevention of illness, use of plant medicines at the beginning of an illness, and a return to homeostasis. We can all benefit from the strengths of herbalism when the need arises.

Conventional medicine is the dominant medical system as practiced by Western physicians. Its use is supported by medical insurance companies, HMOs, physician's associations such as the American Medical Association, and clinical trials. Conventional medicine is based upon the needs of the group, not the individual. The perspective is reductionist, viewing the body as individual physical components and organ systems. This philosophy has created a system of medical specialists such as internists, podiatrists, cardiologists, and urologists.

Conventional medicine shines in traumatic situations such as car accidents, acute infections, medical emergencies, surgical techniques, and in the use of diagnostic machinery. Its emphasis is on treatment after diagnosis and symptom management. We can all benefit from the strengths of conventional medicine when the need arises.

Alternative medical systems are built upon complex systems of theory and practice. Often, these systems have evolved earlier than the conventional medical approach used in the United States, according to the World Health Association. According to the National Institutes of Health (NIH), *complementary medicine* is the adaptation of traditional medicine to the dominant medical system.

Complementary and alternative medicines (CAM) are those healthcare practices not currently considered an integral part of conventional medicine. They include but are not limited to herbs, homeopathy, chiropractic, hypnosis, and acupuncture. According to the NIH, "These practices may lack biomedical explanation, but as they become better researched some…may become widely accepted, whereas others…quietly fade away, yet are important historical footnotes."

Integrative medicine represents an effort to provide a therapeutic model that insists on conventional or alternative medical practices that have received thorough and serious evaluation.

The Language of Folk Medicine

This is an important concept to understand in our discussion on folk medicine. The language, the vocabulary of any folk medicine, such as Southern Folk Medicine, is old as the hills, common to a large portion of the population, and familiar to most of the population within the group or culture. There is no special folk medicine language designed just to be used in special situations. Folk medicines use the everyday language of the everyday peoples, which insures that everyone understands it. Conventional medicine, on the other hand, uses a special language just for doctors, which makes communication difficult between physician and patient and sets physicians apart from their community.

The folk medicine vocabulary and language are intimately woven into the common vernacular of everyday language. In other words, the language of the healers and herbalists is so commonly used that it is difficult for the specific concepts to be conceptualized as a concise folk medicine philosophy by the uninitiated. Sometimes, folk medicine phrases might seem like clichés to those outside the culture. But these sayings speak volumes to those who understand the full depth of the analogies or metaphors.

According to Ruth Trickey, Australian herbalist and author, "In many cultures these concepts become so entwined with the language and a common understanding of health and disease that only a thin line exists between 'commonsense' and the knowledge of the practitioner."

I find this to be very true. For example, if I ask a client, "How are you feeling?" and they answer, "Pretty good," I immediately know that they aren't feeling too well. That they've been having problems of some sort but aren't going to let those problems get them down and are trying to keep a good attitude. I also know that it'll take some pointed questions and a bit of trust before they will fully divulge their health issues. I understand all this from those two simple words.

Across the world, each regional culture has built into the common vocabulary those idioms and phrases that give pages and pages of inferred information…if you understand. In the South, almost everyone knows the meaning of water on the heart, sugar in the blood, high blood, low blood, high blood sugar, holding water, thick blood, and bad blood. These descriptions inherently relay a vast amount of information about health based on their common meanings, but these words and phrases are not acknowledged by the medical community as anything other than colorful phrases that don't really have a medical meaning. Pay attention! What a simple and common communication pathway.

The use of common, ordinary language as a health language is comforting to clients. It helps put them at ease and relaxes any perceived barriers that might exist between client and practitioner. Using the language folks understand helps create trust between client and practitioner, opens lines of communication, and empowers the client with knowledge. The understanding and knowledge then allows the client to fully participate in any decisions regarding their therapeutic protocols. It enables the client to be able to ask important questions regarding their treatment or procedures, or side effects of medications. A common vernacular is a language of support and empowerment.

It's quite easy for common folk to be intimidated by medical language, especially by physicians who use it as a barrier. This limits communication and trust in the therapeutic relationship. It also limits understanding of the health situation by the patient and creates a paternalistic relationship where the physician makes the decisions.

Commonalities of Folk Medicine Systems

Regardless of cultural, religious, or geographical orientation, folk medicine systems from around the world share certain basic, common principles. Given this precept, folk systems can be divided into two broad categories: those whose development, principles, and philosophies were passed in written form, and those which were passed in oral tradition.

Ayurveda, Traditional Chinese Medicine (TCM), and Greek humoral medicine have existed for quite a few thousand years as active forms of healthcare with systemized concepts and principles that were passed to the future in written form. The influence of these three traditions is still widely felt in modern herbalism and in integrative medicine today, especially in the United States, Europe, and Asia.

Other folk traditions, such as Native American practices, Bush medicine, West African Folk Medicine, and other Indigenous systems have also been in existence for quite a few thousand years and developed independently of classical Greek, Ayurvedic, or Traditional Chinese Medicine influences. These folk practices were handed down through oral tradition and developed in isolated pockets based upon the needs of people in those specific, local areas.

Southern and Southern Appalachian Folk Medicine, though in existence for only a few hundred years, evolved to meet the needs of a specific group of people in the American Southeast. It developed from the influence of several different cultures and was traditionally handed down orally from generation to generation. In comparison to TCM or Greek medicine, Southern and Southern Appalachian Folk Medicine are still in their infancy, but, like all folk medicines, continue to evolve.

Luckily, a few others of my generation and I were able to receive these oral traditions from our elders and thus can help ensure its continuance.

Over the years, I've researched and gathered information about folk medicine from a myriad of sources. One of the conclusions I've discerned is that, regardless of location, culture, or orientation, there are common beliefs shared by folk medicine systems around the world. These commonalities are worthy of discussion. While there may be other commonalities among the various types of folk medicine, these are the ones that I have observed.

    ❧   There is an influential force outside of ourselves that is responsible for creation: the first sound, the first dream, the first plant. This force is called God in my neck of the woods, but may be called other names in different cultures and spiritual traditions—Great Spirit or Great Mystery, the Universal Mind, Ancestors, Wheel of Life, Tree of Life, Goddess, Spirits, Elemental Powers, the Force, or a hundred other names depending upon the culture and geographic location.

§ A vital force flows through our bodies, providing energy, motivation, and drive. It also fuels our connection to a higher being and protection against invasion. A strong, vital force signals good health. A diminished or deficient vital force signals poor health or disease. This force may be called ch'i, qi, ki, or prana, but all share a commonality of function or protection for the body. More commonly, it is called Vitality or Vital Energy.

§ The observation of nature is intrinsic to the development of folk systems. People lived very close to the land and depended upon the climate, soil, and the workings of nature in ways that we've forgotten or ignore in our modern, electronic world. The land could be healthy or sickly, dry or wet, cold or hot, and fertile or barren. The language of the land was also the language of health and healing.

§ An understanding of natural laws (using reason) forms the foundation of healing principles. The laws of nature offer general concepts as to why things are the way they are. The laws of nature apply to the entire universe, and they never change. The laws of nature happen independently of us humans. As examples of observable laws of nature: Water flows downhill. Fire spreads across the land. And apples always fall.

§ The state of the world is reflected in the individual. We are only part of the whole, and for this reason, we are not separate from the Earth. What happens to the planet and to the environment affects our health.

§ We are made of the same elements as those of the Earth and are subject to the same laws. The very minerals that form the structure of the Earth form the structure of our bodies. The energy that fueled creation is present at our conception. The fluid that flows across the landscape and gives life to all moves through our bodies, nourishing and cleansing. And the wind that blows across the Earth fills our lungs with breath and brings the rains. We are the children of this planet.

Simple practices of folk medicine developed to assist in the everyday life, health, and prosperity of ordinary people. Our ancestors from the Old World brought healing knowledge, herbs, and health practices from their countries of origin to the New World, using those practices alongside the ones learned from Native Americans. Not all practices that developed in the Old World were useful in the New. The practices that proved useful were kept, and the ones that didn't work were let go. Survival was more important than modality purity.

Even if you are not aware of it, you've probably practiced some type of folk medicine. We have all self-diagnosed, self-treated, used home remedies, and delayed seeking professional medical help. Almost everyone consults their mothers, grandmothers, uncles, friends, pastor, and neighbors about their bothersome aches and pains or other health issues. And what about that internet? Who hasn't looked up their symptoms for a quick assessment? Who hasn't looked up remedies and treatments on the internet once a diagnosis has been made? Who hasn't used special foods or food preparation methods, supplements, prayer, or a lucky object to influence life in some way, whether to heal our bodies or influence the outcome of a situation? My dad carried a buckeye in his pocket for good luck and to stave off arthritis. Some people carry a rabbit's foot or small stone, or light a candle. It's just human nature.

Like the human body, folk medicine is never static, but is continually evolving to meet the health and spiritual needs of the people. The result is a dynamic, whole-body healthcare system able to adapt rapidly to people's needs, a characteristic that makes it the people's medicine. Here in the United States, folk medicine persists not only as a viable modality itself, but has found a niche within mainstream medicine in the protocols, techniques, and philosophies of integrative medicine.

Parental Systems of Southern Folk Medicine

Folk medicine by its very nature should be defined with the community where it is used, especially where oral tradition and local or regional vocabulary defines the concepts and local plant remedies are used. Because the folk medicine of the South is a melding of several different traditions, it shares many of their basic concepts and principles. The same can be said for the Southern and Appalachian accents—they are a combination of several different cultures coming together.

In Southern Folk Medicine, I can certainly see the influence of the humors of Greek medicine, the native plant use of indigenous Southeastern Native Americans, influences from the folk traditions of Northern Europe, specifically of the Irish and Spanish, and influences from both northern and western Africa.

Settlers took what was useful and beneficial, that could improve survival in a harsh, new land, and fused them to make a new system for a new world and a new land.

Each of the parental traditions and systems was manifest with wisdom and knowledge accumulated through centuries of observation, experience, and practice. As a result, you may find the particulars of our folk medicine very familiar if you have studied another folk medicine system. Regardless of the culture, the words to depict the Earth, the elements, and the actions of the climate tend to be described in similar language.

The result of the combination of these systems is a model based on wellness rather than a model based on disease. This is a very important concept. In a harsh land, in a time without antibiotics and modern diagnostic techniques, it was vitally important to stay well. The saying "An ounce of prevention is worth a pound of cure," attributed to Benjamin Franklin, sums up the approach to health in settlement days and one that we would do well to emulate today. A strong body survived; a weak one did not.

In folk systems, there are principles and practices that developed from careful observation of the body—recognizing patterns of dysfunction in disease states. Many diseases and disorders have been around for thousands of years—arthritis, stomach ulcers, sinus infections, abscessed teeth, hernia, malaria, digestive difficulties, colitis, or ovarian cysts to name a few, and over time, tried-and-true methods of treating them have developed which can still be useful today. In a folk system, remedies that work for a disorder are passed to the next generation, and those that don't work are generally ignored, forgotten, or saved for some time in the future when they might be needed.

The Global View

Electronic communications have globalized the world, extending the boundaries of folk medicine past regional, national, and political boundaries. For example, it's very easy for a person in the United States to now be in contact with a traditional

Ayurvedic healer in India. The electronic floodgates are open and herbalists and natural health practitioners from around the world are taking advantage of the opportunities.

People no longer stay in one location their whole lives but move from region to region or country to country, and in the process bring their folk remedies to new areas where there is an exchange of information. You can find acupuncturists in Mississippi, Southern folk herbalists in Chicago, Ayurvedic practitioners in Kansas, Russian folk healers in New York, and Traditional Western herbalists in India. Herbal and other healing techniques are now a cross-cultural exchange with one idiom: If it works, keep it.

One particular example from my practice illustrates this quite well. On this particular day, my first client was a gentleman originally from India complaining of abdominal pain and gas. When I asked what he had been doing to help himself, he replied, "Drinking a cup of hot milk with a spoon of ghee [clarified butter] every night." We discussed his situation, I made some suggestions, and the session ended. My next client was a gentleman originally from England complaining of abdominal pain and gas. I asked what he had been doing for himself. "Drinking a cup of hot milk with a spoon of butter in it every night," he answered. Two different continents, two different men, the same remedy.

Having a culturally diverse clientele helped me to realize that the basic practices of folk medicine are similar regardless of the country of origin, and that in many countries, cross-pollination with other traditions started hundreds if not thousands of years ago. Folk medicine evolved based on the health needs of people, and in general, people's health needs are the same, no matter their culture or geographical location. We all want to be healthy, raise healthy children, do our work well, interact within our communities, and practice our spiritual beliefs. As we continue to expand into a global culture, our folk medicines will continue to evolve, assuming bits and pieces from many different cultures and areas.

Folk Medicine Teaching Methods

Folk medicine has been around as long as humans. The need to take care of ourselves, our families, and the members of our immediate communities and the use of plants in ritual are two major reasons people have sought out herbs and special foods for healing. Though the days of the Granny-healers have largely passed, folk medicine is still alive and well and will continue to evolve, grow, and change to meet our needs.

Traditionally, folk medicine practices were handed down by word of mouth or oral tradition. A master of trade would teach one, maybe two, apprentices over a period of time, generally seven years or longer. Once the apprenticeship was complete, journeyman status was attained and then, with further practice, master of trade or craftsman was achieved. The apprenticeship system is a tried-and-true form of on-the-job training and instruction which developed in Europe during the Middle Ages. In my younger days, it was considered appropriate to call an established herbalist with years of experience, such as Tommie Bass, a Master Herbalist or Master Herbologist. Today, these herbal titles are considered inappropriate and politically incorrect, but they stem from an ancient approach to craftsmanship that served well in its day.

Today, an herbal student might call themselves an apprentice when studying with an established teacher for a few weeks. Or an herbal teacher might offer an apprenticeship of a week, month, or more. The apprenticeship was the first way I learned herbal remedies from my grandparents and, later, Tommie Bass. Ginseng was the primary herb I studied for seven years learning from both my grandmother and father. There are very few herbal students who have the time, the inclination, or the stamina to apprentice for seven years these days.

We have lost a tremendous amount of herbal information because it was never written down. I wish I knew all the information about herbs and plants and how to use them that the old herbalists knew. It can take years of studying with a teacher to fully learn what they have to teach or to understand the nuances of their plant use. Studying with a teacher for a few weeks or months is only the tip of the iceberg.

It saddens me that Native American uses of plants and healing ways are being lost. Keeping to a traditional method of teaching, an elder might only teach one or two students their whole life, and may promise to only teach other Native Americans.

While some teachers may still pass on their learning orally, the process is just as likely to take place in a classroom or other formalized group setting instead of a one-on-one situation. Few teachers follow the more traditional approach of apprenticeship or working with only one student at a time for an extended period. While apprenticeships are still available, teachers more often work with several students concurrently or keep year-round apprenticeship programs open to a variety of students. Internet or distance-learning classes are also available from a wide choice of nontraditional educational institutions such as small herb schools or individual teachers.

In the recent past, folk medicine practices were seen as being confined to the uneducated or those unable to afford conventional medical care. This is certainly not true today. Herbal healing and other forms of folk medicine now appeal to people regardless of socioeconomic level. In my practice, I have consulted with rocket scientists, engineers, university professors, nurses, physicians, ministers, housewives, farmers, teachers, lawyers, physical therapists, psychologists, truck drivers, chicken farmers, and business professionals, all looking for natural ways to approach their health issues or who were looking to build and maintain good health. Folk medicine practices permeate all levels of our society today.

✣ TWO ✣

Common Tenets of Folk Medicine

Part of my ancestry is Cherokee. And in that tradition, you become an adult when you're fifty-two.

—*Alice Walker*

ARTHUR LEE "TOMMIE" BASS (1908–1996) was a blunt, plain-spoken, funny, kind, generous, sentimental, religious, and, truly, all-around good person. The only time I ever heard him speak badly of anyone was to exclaim that, "All politicians are crooks!" No one who ever met Tommie could find fault with his character in any way.

He was and still is, one of the most famous folk herbalists this country ever produced. And luckily, Tommie just lived a short drive away, which made it real easy to visit, study, and learn from this man.

Tommie never married and never learned to drive a car. He often remarked that these two situations relieved him of a lot of stress and contributed to his long life. Tommie had once loved Frankie, the daughter of the landowner whose fields Tommie labored in for much of his adult life. But Frankie had a crippled shoulder and withered arm, which she viewed as an unsightly handicap and an embarrassment. She also had other health issues which led her to forsake any type of romantic relationship. But she and Tommie were close friends until she died, and Tommie never loved anyone else.

Tommie came to the Big Farm in 1937 and lived on the property and worked the owner's fields for payment of rent. Upon the owner's death, Tommie was willed the big house and an acre of land. He never lived in the big house—too many memories and ghosts of his lost love. He did use the kitchen for cooking and bathroom for hygiene, but preferred his shack for sleeping and herbal work.

Tommie began his woods training at the tender age of four by helping his father gather ginseng and other wild herbs for market. By the age of six, he was working in the cotton fields helping to pick cotton. Tommie often remarked that it didn't matter the skin color, "we all had to sharecrop." By the age of eight, Tommie was at the logging mill peeling bark for crossties. He soon graduated to helping his father fur trap and gather herbs on a full-time basis. He made enough money from trapping muskrat, skunk, mink, beaver, fox, and raccoon to buy his winter clothes, hunting and trapping supplies, and a few groceries.

He never went to proper school but was taught to read by his mother from the Bible and the Blue-Back Speller. Both his mother and father were herbalists, a tradition that ran in the Bass family from England, and Tommie often remarked that his parents, "knew so much about how the body worked that they could have been doctors."

In addition to gathering herbs and working with his father, Tommie began working with Aunt Molly Kirby, a black herbist and midwife down the mountain from where his family lived. Aunt Molly became too old and slow to traipse along the mountain ridges, and so she employed Tommie to help gather the herbs she needed in her practice. Over the next few years, Tommie learned much about gathering and using native herbs from her.

All told, Tommie began hunting herbs in earnest about the age of nine and didn't stop until well into his eighties.

As one of my influential teachers, Tommie lived eighty-eight years and most of those years were spent learning about herbs and helping people. Tommie didn't believe in cures, but rather sought to help support the natural processes of the body. The exception to this philosophy was his skin cancer salve, which Tommie truly believed was an effective topical remedy.

Tommie never charged for an herbal consultation but did sell herbs to his clients. No one was ever turned away due to lack of money, and he gave away as many herbs as he sold. A consult with Tommie was an adventure. He was likely to entertain you by quoting poetry, singing a song, or playing the harmonica. For Tommie, people coming for herbal aid was a social event as well as a healing one.

He considered himself an herbist whose main job in life was bringing ease to those in need. Tommie usually saw around five or six people on average a day, but as his practice grew there might be ten or more to arrive for his help at any time. He didn't take appointments; people just arrived and waited their turn. In the 1970s, the local paper, *The Gadsden Times,* ran several articles about his life and work which increased his business tremendously. By 1980, Tommie was seeing about 2,000 people a year, mostly poor African-Americans and poor whites who had no health insurance or money to pay a doctor.

In 1985, the *Wall Street Journal* ran a front-page essay about him. This was followed by a double-volume scholarly look at his life and herb use by John Crellin and Jane Philpott, *A Reference Guide to Medicinal Plants* and *Trying to Give Ease* published by Duke University. There were also several popular books, one by Darryl Patton, *Mountain Medicine: The Herbal Remedies of Tommie Bass,* a couple of documentaries, and even more newspaper articles. Tommie Bass, who never learned to drive, became the most well-known folk herbalist in the country.

In addition to the people who made the trip to Shinbone Ridge to see Tommie, many others would simply mail him a letter stating their symptoms and asking for herbs. He answered every single letter, mailed folks the herbs, and hoped for some sort of payment in return. As Tommie's reputation spread, new clientele arrived who were able to pay in cash money. These folks were well-educated and would visit their physician and then visit the herbist. Tommie felt that doctors do a "good job with what they've got to work with," and that someday, "they will find out about herbs and do their job a bit better." But fame didn't change Tommie at all, and he never took advantage of those who could pay the big money.

He had strong opinions on health and never hesitated to relay those opinions. Tommie would show a client where to find the needed herb in the woods, how to harvest it, and how to cook it up. It was quite an adventure to be Tommie's client. At the very least, you left with a bag of dried herbs and directions on how to cook them. As the years passed, fewer and fewer people were willing to cook up the herbs themselves, too busy or "too lazy" as Tommie said, and either relied upon him to make the brews or bought encapsulated products. This became so common that in his mid-seventies, Tommie switched to using over-the-counter products, believing that "at least they were getting down some help."

Tommie sold his popular cancer salve to individual clients, at trade day flea markets, and in shops around the local area. The basic salve recipe came from his English grandparents who had made Bass's Salve in England and modified it for the available herbs found in the Southeast. The primary ingredients were pine tar, wild tobacco, summer cedar, and black walnut or slippery elm bark. Sometimes yellow sulfur was added to boost efficiency. The oil base was either hog lard or beef tallow. The salve was used on any type of skin spot, skin cancer, or bed sores, and for hemorrhoids, as well as cracked skin.

In addition to Bass's Salve, Tommie's other popular herbal product was his cough syrup. This compound formula contained a number of local plants, and the recipe often changed with availability of herbs. One of his favorite recipes for coughs and colds was wild cherry bark, sweetgum bark or leaves, boneset, red root, mullein, yellowroot, rabbit tobacco, and sumac. Sometimes he also added calamus, bugleweed, or skullcap. The herbs were decocted for about twenty minutes, strained, and then sugar was added to make a syrup. Another favorite cough remedy was wild cherry bark, sweetgum bark, slippery elm bark, and mullein leaves.

For rheumatism, Tommie used cucumber magnolia, dogwood bark, prickly ash, skullcap, and bay. He viewed formulas as herbs "working like a team to get the job done." But as a true Southern herbalist, Tommie also used whatever substances were available that would work whether it was an herb or not. His liniment rub was composed of green rubbing alcohol, vinegar, ammonia, camphor gum, and turpentine. This was all mixed in a jar to sit overnight. He sold it for years to use on bee stings, poison ivy, and rheumatism, and it worked amazingly well.

Before the popularity of milk thistle, Tommie recommended either wild cherry bark or red oak bark for nonspecific problems with the liver or those symptoms brought on by a "chill on the liver." This would include pain on the right side and a certain feeling of hardness on palpitation. Later, he did use milk thistle and felt it was effective. He also recommended topical herbal poultices and a heating pad on the liver to help break the chill.

For diabetes and other endocrine problems, Tommie used Queen Anne's lace, Queen of the Meadow (also known as Joe Pye or gravel root), red root, or huckleberry. In combination with skullcap, passionflower or blue vervain, the herbs for high sugar could also help with high blood pressure because the two disorders were so often found together.

Over his lifespan, Tommie saw herbal medicine change from an almost forgotten vocation to an active profession. Although his practice changed with the times, the reality of who Tommie Bass was never did. Fame didn't diminish him. He stayed devoted to his community, accessible and open to his clients, and nonjudgmental and personable in session. When he passed, a huge depository of traditional herbal knowledge passed with him. I miss Tommie, but I'm also proud of the influence his teachings have had on my life and profession.

Similarities of Folk Medicine Systems

In folk medicine, there are no magic bullets, no quick fixes, and no instant cures. Coaxing the body into lifestyle habits takes time, energy, and a willingness to make those lifestyle changes. Understanding the directing principles of folk medicine can provide guidelines for making those changes. Tommie Bass used to say, "A person will change when they don't have a choice. And that's when they get desperate and think they're gonna die." Doesn't it make more sense to change unhealthy behaviors before desperation sets in?

Generally, the tenets of folk medicine were passed orally within teachings or were so common that they were inferred and understood by all. The tenets provide a framework for good health practices that are common to many folk systems.

The following tenets were developed from various sources, including: oral teachings I learned; my own personal experience in clinical practice; observations of indigenous practices; and principles of folk medicine published by McGill Molson Medical Informatics in 2000; and from Research Council on Complementary Medicine in Great Britain.

The tenets of folk medicine are so important that each one deserves its own book. I sincerely encourage you to further investigate any that speak to you or pique your interest. Books, articles, and research methods can be found regarding each one.

1. **HEALTH IS A POSITIVE STATE, THE RIGHT OF EACH INDIVIDUAL, AND A CONTINUALLY EVOLVING PROCESS.**   We all have a basic right to pursue good health. It goes along with the pursuit of happiness. Good health should not be dependent upon health insurance companies, Congressional approval, or the result of a political agenda. It should be an inalienable right with equal access by everyone and the primary focus of spiritual, political, educational, and economic organizations and institutions.

Healthy people make wise choices. Healthy people take an active role in their families, communities, and country. Healthy brains work better, think better, create better. And healthy people raise healthy children. Healthy people are less likely to make decisions based on fear. Healthy people are more likely to make healthy lifestyle choices that maintain their health.

"If you've got your health, you've got everything." How many times have you heard that saying? The trouble is, folks often don't value their health until a crisis strikes. And then it could be too late. Mickey Mantle best summed it up: "If I'd known I was gonna live this long, I'd have taken a lot better care of myself."

Self-care leads to good physical, mental, and emotional health. It's a habit that must be cultivated until it becomes part of your family culture. If you rush around, never feed your children a home-cooked meal, and never take the time for relaxing activities for yourself or your children, then that's what you are teaching them—the habit of a rushed life and take-out food. Not a scenario that encourages good health habits. The key to changing this view of health is education, education, education.

2. WE HAVE A DUTY TO PURSUE GOOD HEALTH.   The mind, body, emotions, and spirit are not separate, but integrated to complete who we are. In order to be the very best we can be, in order to achieve our highest potential, we must be healthy in all levels of our existence. The body is the temple, the physical housing of spirit on Earth, and what we do to the body, we do to the temple and ultimately to the soul. This sacrament between God and humans is well-known but not well-followed. This sacrament must also extend to the very Earth on which we depend for life. If the body is the temple of the soul, then the Earth is the temple of the body.

We also have a duty to our children, our grandchildren, and the future generations. We are their seed, their progenitors. Their health depends upon our health. If we live lives of stress, trauma, and poor nutrition, then that's the seed we are casting forth.

3. THE BODY HAS INHERENT SELF-REGULATORY MECHANISMS THAT CAN BE SUPPORTED BY TRADITIONAL THERAPIES.   Health is a continually evolving process; it is never finished. "Constance of the internal environment is the condition for free and independent life," said Claude Bernard (1813–1878), a French physiologist and contemporary of Pasteur whose works in experimental medicine are best associated with the concept of homeostasis. Bernard taught that the body maintains a constant internal environment by many continual and compensatory reactions which restore a state of equilibrium in response to any outside changes. In this way, the human body maintains independence from the external environment.

In 1926, Walter Bradford Cannon first coined the term *homeostasis* to mean the stability of the inner world of the human body. He believed that the brain coordinates the body systems to maintain a set of points considered healthiest. Either internal or external disturbances can threaten homeostasis, and sometimes those threats are large enough to create deviations from the set points. When threats do occur, the nervous and hormonal systems induce emotional and action states that result in observable changes in behavior. These changes, which are crucial for the body to self-regulate, help trigger a return to homeostasis. If homeostasis is poorly regulated, disease or damage to the body may result.

Ultimately, it's all about homeostasis, how our body maintains a stable internal environment. Our body works hard to maintain homeostasis or our good health—really hard. As the body struggles with chronic illness, its definition of homeostasis slowly changes. At each point of physical degradation, our body learns a new level of set points. This is one reason why a diagnosis of stage 4 cancer can be so surprising. As one client put it, "I'd been feeling just fine until last week when I got sick and my wife made me go to the doctor." After a series of tests, this client was diagnosed with cancer in every major organ system and only lived a few weeks. His body worked really hard at maintaining homeostasis up until the very end.

Traditional therapies shine at helping the body return to homeostasis or helping maintain homeostasis. Healthy foods, exercise, herbs, movement, massage, and other natural health techniques have stood the test of time in supporting good health.

4. **THE BODY IS NEVER STATIC, EVEN IN HEALTH, WHICH RESULTS IN A HOMEODYNAMIC ORGANISM CONTINUALLY ADAPTING TO NEW STATES OF BEING.** The human body is continually adapting, building, and rebuilding, always in a constant state of activity even when we are asleep. We are constantly creating new cells and disposing of old ones, repairing damaged tissues, cleansing toxins, releasing hormones, digesting food, thinking, blinking, and dreaming. Fluids constantly circulate around the

body, neurons fire unceasingly, and our senses are always on alert. Heart and breath never stop. We are an energy system in perpetual motion.

Our bodies are continually monitoring and coordinating these responses in an effort to maintain homeostasis, to minimize any disturbance in the body. The human body works hard at ensuring that when changes do occur, they are small and stay within narrow limits. In this way, homeostasis actively responds to subtle ebbs and flows of fluids, electrolytes, gases, and sugars at a working temperature of about 98.6°F, which is considered optimal for enzyme functioning.

In 1988, Sterling and Eyer proposed the theory of allostasis, a concept of homeostasis not concerned with subtle ebbs and flows, but rather one that responds to a challenge instead. Allostasis is an adaptive response that factors in the roles of the endocrine system, the autonomic nervous system and various hormones such as adrenalin, cortisol, testosterone, estrogen, and various neurotransmitters. This is our reaction to acute stress.

In the long term, however, continual allostatic overload can lead to nervous exhaustion, chronic disease, chronic fatigue, endocrine disorders, heart disease, and other chronic illnesses. Chronic stress, regardless of the cause, places us in survival mode where our problems or life situations become the supreme focus of our daily existence and the instrument which decreases vital energy levels. As long as we are in survival mode, living in fear and apprehension, we cannot heal rapidly or fully; both health and happiness are elusive. As long as we are in survival mode, we don't make wise decisions, but instead react without thinking. Our duty is to move out of survival mode, toward health and into higher functioning.

5. GOOD DIGESTION IS THE BASIS OF GOOD HEALTH.   Since the time of Hippocrates, a strong digestive capacity has been seen as vital to good health. The ability to assimilate life-giving nutrients is the foundation of our well-being. "All diseases begin in the gut," was one of the first axioms I learned in my training. At first glance, this statement may sound foolish. But upon deeper investigation, its truth emerges.

About 60 percent to 70 percent of the immune system resides in the gut, and about 80 percent of antibody-secreting cells reside in the gut mucosa. Just think about this for a moment. Each time we eat, our immune system must cope with foreign invaders such as phytochemicals, bacteria, food additives, dyes, and unhealthy oils. Food itself, though nourishing, is also considered a foreign invader by our immune systems. In light of this, you can see how our immune systems can become hijacked by digestive issues.

Eating is a life-giving process that should be nourishing for the mind, body, and spirit. Nowadays, folks take eating for granted, cramming meals into busy schedules without taking the time to enjoy the meal or to rest and digest after it. People eat too fast, eat while driving, and eat on the go. It's a reason so many Americans suffer from some type of digestive difficulty such as bloating, gas, and abdominal pain or inflammation, or even irritable bowel syndrome. Eating poor-quality food is another.

Digestion is individual. Some people have iron digestive systems that seem to be able to handle any type of food, while others lack the ability to digest even the gentlest of foods.

For its own health, the digestive tract relies upon probiotics, the good bacteria that live in the digestive tract, along with digestive enzymes and a strong mucosa lining as crucial lines of defense against illness. If the digestive system is overwhelmed by bacteria-laden food, poor-quality food, stress, or food sensitivities, the immune system itself becomes damaged. This not only leads to a myriad of bowel disorders, but also to the highjacking of the immune system and, ultimately, the nutritional failure of the system. If the immune system in our gut is constantly busy with digestive problems, then its attention isn't focused on fighting off infection, killing invaders, or eating cancer cells.

6. IN MANY INSTANCES, THE BODY CAN HEAL ITSELF IF GIVEN THE RIGHT TOOLS.   Rest and relaxation, nutritious food, healing herbs, gentle movement, sweating, sunlight, clean air and water, laughter, meditation or prayer, being with family and friends, and stress-relief techniques are just a few of the tools for good living and repairing our health. They really don't require extraordinary measures to achieve, but commitment and dedication in their pursuit.

Fortunately, natural medicine offers many modalities upon which to draw for good health. Herbalism, aromatherapy, massage, Tai Chi, yoga, nutritional supplements, guided imagery, acupressure, acupuncture, special foods and diets, juicing, energy work such a Reiki or therapeutic touch, homeopathy, various exercise modalities, deep breathing, music, art, and dance therapy, psychological counseling, biofeedback, deep breathing techniques, Alexander Technique, Feldenkrais Technique, light therapy, and many more modalities. The majority of these do not have scientific studies to validate their use; all you can do is try and see if it helps.

But healing is never certain—can never be guaranteed. There are no promises of good health, not by traditional medicine and not by conventional medicine. We just do the best we can. I've seen people who have never smoked but have lung cancer; those that have never drank alcohol, but have cirrhosis of the liver; and those that eat healthy and well but have colon cancer. We can only plod along and do our best, and that includes giving our bodies the proper tools to do its job.

7. **BUILDING A HEALTHY INTERNAL TERRAIN SHOULD BE THE PRIMARY GOAL OR FOCUS OF FOOD AND HERBAL THERAPIES.**   Louis Pasteur (1822–1895) believed that microbes bore unique responsibility for disease and fermentation, while his counterpart Claude Bernard held that the disturbed functioning of an organism creates an environment in which microbes cause illness. During his lifetime, Pasteur argued that dealing with illness requires attacking with chemical medicines from outside the body, as well as vaccinations. Bernard, on the other hand, maintained that a healthy organism was the best defense against sickness. There is something to be said for both viewpoints.

A healthy, internal terrain also includes positive thoughts, feelings, and emotions. If our emotions are unbalanced, our thoughts negative, and our relationships stressful, then how can we be healthy? Resentment, fear, worry, and jealousy affect our internal terrain and impair our health as much as any physical invader. Conflict and strife within our families, our places of work, and our communities create stress, which sabotages good health. Maintaining good relationships with self, family, and community is a vital aspect of Southern and Appalachian Folk Medicine and these relationships are considered preventive measures for avoiding illness.

8. **A VITAL OR LIFE FORCE PERMEATES ALL LIVING CELLS.**   Whether it is referred to as the innate intelligence of the cell, as Vital Energy, ch'i, or

heavenly power, it is the force which is present during life and missing in death. The concept of the vital force has its roots in the teachings of Hippocrates (400 BCE) and of Galen (190 BCE), who defined it as innate to the human constitution. Paracelsus (1493–1541) viewed it as an active, directing intelligence which maintained and repaired the organism in a dynamic fashion. George Stahl (1660–1734), a German physicist and chemist, believed that matter was spirit in motion and was divided into two categories: organic and inorganic. He further believed that all parts of the body were passive and could only be activated or moved by the release of energy from the soul. The soul uses the chemical processes of the body for this release. Death, he reasoned, is the departure of the vital force or the exiting of the soul (*Life Itself: Exploring the Realm of the Living Cell*, Rensberger, B., p. 6, 1998).

Regardless of whether it is called the Vital Force, ch'i, prana, or ki, almost every culture in the world defines and describes this concept.

The source of our energy is, of course, mitochondria. Those little powerhouses create ATP, a form of chemical energy that every cell can use. Mitochondria has its own DNA separate from our forty-six chromosomes. We inherit our mitochondria DNA from our mothers. And while mitochondria can, by no means, be defined as our soul, the description of their activities certainly parallels ancient writings.

9. **SYMPTOMS ARE VIEWED AS THE BODY'S MESSENGERS AND SHOULD NOT BE SUPPRESSED UNNECESSARILY.**   Vital energy is a complex mechanism that functions both as a defense system and an internal intelligence which protects the body from invasion, supervises the actions of the internal organs, and monitors the reactions of the mind. Within this purview, vital energy becomes a complex interaction between mind and emotions, nervous system, immune system, and mitochondria. Symptoms are a response of the body's defense mechanism. Stahl, for instance, viewed fevers, hemorrhages, and palpitations as natural reactions by an intelligent and harmonious body confronting some stress. One must therefore respect these symptoms: They are the *self-healing* efforts of the body.

This doesn't mean that folks who are ill shouldn't be as comfortable as possible. No one wants to be in pain. It's hard to think and function when in pain, and it drains our energy, causing fatigue. Pain itself can raise blood pressure. Pain-relieving and anti-inflammatory remedies can help keep a person functional, going to work and taking care of business. Obviously, this doesn't mean that life-saving drugs shouldn't be administered when necessary. Of course they should: If you need insulin, then take insulin.

But it does mean that suppressing symptoms does not necessarily provide any healing benefit. A person can faithfully take their diabetes medication and their blood sugar may appear to be under control, but damage can still be happening. Blood pressure can still rise and kidney damage can still occur. However, if that same person took their prescription, noninsulin diabetes medication, followed a healthy diet plan, exercised regularly, reduced stress, and slept well, the potential for reducing or alleviating any damage would be tremendous.

Even scarier, you only have to watch the latest prescription drug commercials on television to realize the potential of damage from medications. The side effects for some drugs are often more debilitating than the disease itself. Natural approaches, such as using herbs and foods, have fewer side effects, and the ones present are generally mild.

10. THE BODY IS VIEWED AND TREATED AS WHOLE: MIND, BODY, AND SPIRIT.   One part of the body cannot be affected without impacting the whole organism. Any treatment that alters a part changes the whole. From this point of view, true reductionism is only useful if viewed within the whole; otherwise it can lead to incomplete explanations.

Can the true nature of the forest be understood by studying only one tree? In the same vein, how much can you tell about the health of the body by just studying one organ system? We are the sum of our parts. We must view the body with an awareness of all parts and the intricate dance that happens between these parts. Just to be fair, from a practical point of view, it is extremely difficult to take into account every possible influence upon a person's health. We can only do our best.

Even thinking of the human body as a physical, emotional, mental, and spiritual being is a bit reductionist. The concept of holism reunites the various planes of our existence into an integrated whole.

11. TRADITIONAL THERAPIES EMPHASIZE PREVENTION.   It is easier to forestall an illness than to treat it. Preventive health aims at reducing risk factors for chronic illness through lifestyle alterations and changes. For example, by emphasizing good nutrition with attention to eating foods high in antioxidants and other phytochemicals, maintaining a healthy weight, getting adequate rest and exercise, and reducing the impact of stress, traditional approaches to health can head off illness before it strikes, or can reduce its impact or shorten its length if it does strike.

These same preventive health approaches can help shorten the time in old age when a person declines, helping that person to live an active, full life into old age rather than spending their last years immobile or in a nursing home. Consequently, we have to view preventive health as more than just medical screenings and examinations; it is the support and nurturing of the self.

Our current Western conventional medicine places no emphasis on preventive medicine. The United States has the most expensive healthcare system in the world, but is very ineffective at keeping people well. It's true that the United States doesn't have price control on drugs, and the high cost of drugs certainly increases healthcare costs. But that's not the only reason. Other reasons for the high cost of healthcare in the U.S. are the use of expensive diagnostic technology, the high cost of administration, and the inability of the government to be able to buy drugs in bulk quantity.

But most influential on the cost of healthcare is the lack of emphasis on preventive health practices that could forestall a chronic illness until later in life or indefinitely. Traditional therapies support preventive practices that extend healthy, active living into the elder years. Once again, it boils down to education, education, education.

12. TRADITIONAL THERAPIES SHOULD BE NONTOXIC AND NONINVASIVE, EXCEPT IN ACUTE OR EMERGENCY SITUATIONS. Traditional remedies and therapies support the body through nutritive action; the building of a healthy internal terrain; a specific action upon an organ or body system; and by supporting individual constitutions or by helping achieve emotional or spiritual health.

Strong, toxic remedies are confined to the venue of conventional medicine where side effects can be monitored. Strong, potentially toxic herbs should only be used by experienced herbalists in extreme situations, and used only in low doses, by the drop, as appropriate to the condition.

13. THERE IS A SPECIFIC PLANT TO REMEDY EACH ILLNESS.   Folk healers understand the gift of the plants and the healing benefits inherent in their properties. Cherokee medicine men, African-American root healers, Appalachian herbalists, Bush healers, and other folk healers share the common belief that there is a plant for every illness. Tommie Bass believed that "God made the world with all the plants and the fishes in the sea. He did all this before he made anybody to take care of the world....We were made from the earth and we've got to go back to the earth to get something to make our bodies tick. We are part of the earth."

One Native American tale teaches how humans got medicine. To make a long story short, humans had become overbearing and aggressive and were destroying the Earth. The animals got together and determined that to save the Earth, humans must die. After trying several ways to kill humans but not having much success, the tiniest, littlest creatures upon the Earth, the ones you can't see and which are invisible, volunteered to invade humans and kill them from the inside. After many days of sickness, a great cry came upon the land from the humans. The cry was so loud the animals couldn't escape the sound. Finally, the Green People (plants) could take no more and agreed to help humans so that they might grow and take their place in the council. The Green People stepped forward and vowed that for every illness created by the invisible beings, a plant would offer the remedy.

14. IT WILL TAKE AWHILE TO GET BETTER. WE NEED TO CONVALESCE.   Generally, folks don't contract chronic illnesses overnight and therefore won't get better overnight. Years of living or working in stressful situations or having a stressful family life, years of being around chemical fumes or noxious odors, of drinking polluted water and eating factory-farmed fruits and commercial vegetables and meats, and breathing polluted air, take a toll on the body. To fully heal, a person must step away from the very situation and factors that caused the illness and find a situation or place that offers rest and healing.

HOW HUMANS RECEIVED MEDICINE,
AS TOLD BY DAVID WINSTON

The Cherokee legend of how people got medicine also confirms the belief that we are part of the Earth and can't separate ourselves from it. In the short version, man had overrun the Earth, polluting air and waters and destroying the land, rendering it incapable of producing healthy food or life. Mankind was selfishly killing the plants and animals for personal gain, disregarding the welfare of all who lived upon the Earth. The animals held council to determine what might be done to resolve the problem, to stop the damage to the Earth before it was rendered unfit for all life. After many days of meeting, the bears decided they would take care of the problem by killing mankind.

Because bears walk upon two legs and make use of their paws like hands, it was decided they would fashion a bow and arrow to kill mankind. One old bear volunteered his life for the making of the bow, offering his guts for the string. Another bear offered to deliver the fatal blow. When the time came to kill mankind, the bear found his paws did not function the same as hands, and he could not pull the bowstrings. In disgrace, he reported to the council and offered to cut off his paws to better pull the bow. But the leader of the council opposed the action, saying that to maim oneself to better kill would make the bear no better than mankind.

In despair, the animals held another council to discuss how best to rid the land of mankind.

After many days of meeting, the smallest animals came forward. These animals were so tiny they couldn't be seen. "We'll take care of the humans," they said. These tiny animals invaded mankind through their food and water, through the air and sky. This caused mankind great pain and affliction. A great cry went up upon the land. It was the cry of mankind suffering and dying. This cry went on for many days until finally the plants could stand it no longer. Out of pity for mankind, the plants, the Green People, came forward. "We take pity on you," they said. "For each affliction, we will provide a remedy. From this day forward, for each disease, a plant will step forward to provide a cure."

Often we don't recognize the early signs of dysfunction in the body and so live with nagging aches and pains, digestive difficulties, and feeling not quite ourselves for many years before a definitive diagnosis is reached. A physician once remarked to me that it takes about five years from the time the first symptoms appear until markers show in blood work for many chronic disorders. That's five years or longer of living with discomfort, uncertainty, and pain. That's five years the body has worked really, really hard to maintain homeostatic functioning. And that's five years that folks may be told that their symptoms "are all in their head" because blood tests aren't conclusive.

Convalescence is a word that doesn't often make it into our health vocabulary. It is the action of recovery after illness, including the time it takes to manifest the recovery. Convalescence is a gradual process; unhealthy behaviors need to be replaced by healthy behaviors and the damage to the internal organs repaired. Multiple modalities, such as herbs, nutrition, bodywork, and prayer, may be needed to aid the repair of the body and recovery of health.

15. LIFESTYLE HAS A MAJOR IMPACT ON HEALTH.   There is no doubt that lifestyle impacts health. Medical journals routinely publish studies on just this topic. Poor eating habits, poor-quality food, lack of exercise, smoking, excessive consumption of alcohol, poverty, and poor hygiene all affect our quality of health. And let's not forget the effects of stress and emotional trauma.

The folks I've met who have truly recovered from a chronic illness are the ones who were willing to make major changes in their lives. Making these types of major changes is hard to do, especially with a family. Our beliefs, attitudes, and egos become bound up in the very behaviors that are often the most damaging to our health and, sometimes, our family culture. This makes it extremely difficult to give up those behaviors because, on some level, we believe that we are who we are because of them, or that our family won't accept us if we change our behaviors. I once had a smoker tell me that he would never give up smoking because he wouldn't be the same person if he did, and he liked who he was. A wife once told me that she couldn't change the way she cooked, from unhealthy to healthy, because her husband and kids would be mad, even though those food choices were contributing to their obesity.

Lifestyle is actually the part of living over which we have some control. For example, the International Agency for Research on Cancer (IARC) issued a report in 2014 that discussed the lifestyle behaviors that lead to an increased risk of cancer—smoking tobacco, drinking alcohol, overweight/obesity, and lack of exercise. These are lifestyle behaviors based on choices made. We can choose to change those behaviors—we have choice.

16. THE CAUSE OF ILLNESS, NOT JUST THE SYMPTOMS, SHOULD BE FOUND AND TREATED. Folk healers and herbalists are good detectives seeking to find the cause of illness. By seeking the source, by peeling back the layers of illness, recovery can begin.

Native American healers and later Southern folk herbalists, like Granny Light, Tommie Bass, and John Lee, an African-American healer from North Carolina, classified illnesses into two categories: natural and supernatural. Natural illnesses were further divided into physical and psychological disorders. Physical illnesses include invasion by microbes, trauma, exposure to toxins, poor nutrition, and chronic infections. Psychological illnesses include the effects of stress, nervous breakdown, worry, depression, emotional conflict related to personal relationships, and mental disturbances. Today, supernatural or spiritual illnesses might include addiction, evil acts and behaviors, or any behavior that takes you away from your ethical center. In the old days, this might also include possession by spirits, hexes, and other magical acts.

Understanding the source of illness expands remedy options and brings peace of mind to the sick. People want to know, "Why am I sick? Have I done something to cause this? Where did this come from? Why is this happening to me?" Sometimes a cause or source of affliction can be traced, such as a car accident years earlier, or an illness, such as a virus, which never seemed to go away. But sometimes, there are no answers to these questions. Sometimes we just have to say, "I don't know what caused it, but let's see if we can find out." And then the important question, "When did your illness begin and what was happening in your life prior to that time?"

Natural health techniques and conventional medicine are not mutually exclusive; they can be used together in an integrative fashion for the benefit of those in need. Finding ground where we can all work together in mutual respect will be vitally important for the health of this country in the future.

17. TRAUMA, EMOTIONAL DISTRESS, AND STRESS ARE MAJOR CAUSES OF DISEASE.   Clinical research and case studies too numerous to mention clearly make the connection between stress and our health. Chronic stress engages both psychological and physiological processes resulting in lowered immune functioning, fatigue, and lack of vitality and drive. The longer the stress continues, the less we are engaged in the joy of living. Every activity becomes a chore and fatigue the constant companion. Chronic stress, emotional distress, and trauma increase risk factors for all chronic diseases including cardiovascular disease, diabetes, cancer, fibromyalgia, chronic fatigue, and autoimmune disorders.

Stress and trauma can increase or decrease the appetite. It can cause digestive difficulties such as heartburn and constipation or diarrhea, and affect blood sugar levels. Chronic stress can cause a racing heartbeat, heart palpitations, and contribute to high blood pressure. It can cause poor sleep quality, mood changes, depression, and muscular aches and pains, especially in the lower back. Chronic stress can affect fertility and a woman's monthly cycle. And chronic stress impacts the activity of the immune system.

Post-traumatic stress disorder (PTSD) is a debilitating form of chronic stress that occurs whenever someone has experienced the sudden death of a loved one, war, rape, or robbery, or has been part of a natural disaster, to name a few examples. Women are more than twice as likely as men to experience PTSD, and children can experience it also. In addition to the previously mentioned symptoms, people with PTSD may also experience nightmares, flashbacks, and unwanted memories of the event.

18. CHRONIC ILLNESSES MAY INVOLVE COMPLEX PATTERNS AND MULTI-ORGAN SYSTEMS, AND CANNOT BE ADEQUATELY ASSESSED BY STANDARD MEDICAL TESTS.   As discussed earlier, by the time blood work shows the effects of fibromyalgia, the average sufferer may have been symptomatic for about five years. Pain and suffering, a feeling of wrongness in the body, and a desire for help are too often diagnosed as "nerves" or "all in the head" or "stress." And too often the physician prescribes an antidepressant or antianxiety drug which doesn't fix the problem and may even create different ones. It is within this five years that improved nutrition, herbs, and lifestyle changes can impact the illness or even totally head it off at the pass.

Folk healers look and listen to the individual and make assessments based upon patterns of dysfunction in the body. These patterns can be discerned by completing an assessment based upon signs found in the nails, tongue, face, hair, and pulse, understanding the client's symptoms, listening to their life story, and asking targeted questions.

In Southern and Appalachian Folk Medicine, certain constitutions may have certain health tendencies. Knowing a person's constitution can provide a direction for the assessment process. By understanding which disorders a particular constitution might be prone to, a person can make targeted lifestyle changes, improve their diet, and utilize appropriate herbs. This will be discussed in greater detail under the individual constitutions and their elements.

19. AN INDIVIDUAL WITH A CHRONIC DISORDER MAY NOT EXHIBIT THE SAME SYMPTOMS AS ANOTHER INDIVIDUAL WITH THE SAME DISORDER.   Chronic disorders have a way of being individually symptomatic. For example, one person with hypothyroidism may gain weight while another may not. One person with allergies may experience rashes while another may have a runny nose. One person with fibromyalgia may experience chronic muscle aches and pains while another may feel fatigue and depression.

Men have an increased risk for cardiovascular disease than women. Early studies of heart disease focused on unhealthy social behaviors in which men participated but women didn't. During these studies, male symptoms of heart disease were fully documented, especially that of heart attack, and it was assumed that women exhibited the same symptoms during an attack. However, more recent studies (2003) show that men and women may have totally different symptoms during a heart attack and that about 50 percent of women don't experience chest pain during an attack.

Women are often ignored in medical research. When we think about the fact that women are more likely than men to have a chronic disease, this becomes mind-boggling. The very population most prone to chronic disease is the least studied for chronic disease. Women are more likely to die from cardiovascular disease than men. Nonsmoking women are more likely to have lung cancer than men. Women are more likely to have depression than men. But in the majority of clinical studies, women make up less than one-third of the subjects. Fortunately, traditional folk systems focus on the individual and look for patterns of dysfunction rather than medical diagnosis, as we'll discuss in the next tenet.

20. EACH PERSON IS UNIQUE AND INDIVIDUAL; THEREFORE, PROTOCOLS SHOULD BE INDIVIDUALIZED.   Traditional remedies and healing protocols are not one-size-fits-all. Since we are all unique individuals with our own constitutions, our healing programs should be just as unique. A remedy that might work brilliantly for one person might only work so-so for another, or not at all. A remedy or healing plan should be designed for the individual, not for the masses.

We all have different bodies, different personalities, and different ways of handling life. We have different stressors and different situations at home. Recognizing that the body is more than a physical entity, but also an emotional, mental, and spiritual one, we must take into account how different personalities handle life, stress, and ill-health. We must also take into account that each gender is a unique cocktail of hormones and that affects mind, body, and spirit.

We all have individual constitutions, and our disorders will manifest as individually as ourselves. A foundation of folk medicine is the acknowledgment that remedies must be individualized to be most effective. A one-size-fits-all approach to medicine is the purview of conventional medicine and backbone of the pharmaceutical industry, but is not always the best approach.

21. INDIVIDUALS MUST TAKE AN ACTIVE ROLE IN MAINTAINING THEIR OWN HEALTH.   Individual responsibility and accountability are paramount for good health and longevity. We must be responsible for ourselves, learn all we can about preventative health, and take steps to implement self-care measures that support and nourish our minds, bodies, and spirits. In doing so, we also become examples for our families, neighbors, and communities.

Sometimes how we need to take care of ourselves, what we need to do to be healthy, is opposed by our family culture. Whenever we eat differently, sleep differently, stop smoking, stop drinking sodas or alcohol, or release any behavior that is not supporting our health and happiness, family members may feel threatened. They may feel that our new behavior is distancing us from them or that we feel that we are "better" than they are. All we can do is ask for the support of our family and friends when making lifestyle changes. Often by explaining our process to them and asking for their support, they will come on board. They may not understand our decisions, but love can overcome their trepidations.

22. OUR CULTURE INFLUENCES OUR HEALTH.   The South is one of the few areas in the country with a cultural identity still intact, though this influence is not always reflected in a positive health manner. Currently, the South has the highest rate in the United States of both obesity and type 2 diabetes, and cultural influences play a huge role in these statistics. Eating fast food is considered all-American, patriotic, and pretty cool. It is less expensive and less time-consuming than cooking at home. This makes for poor nutrition choices.

Regardless of the area of the country in which we live, cultural differences must be taken into account in healthcare management. Cultural attitudes and norms are handed down within microcultures from one generation to the next. When we assume that everyone must conform to the norms of the dominant culture or that everyone has conformed, this only guarantees that many subgroups and minority classes fall through the cracks.

In addition to the dominant Caucasian culture, other large cultural groups in this country include African-Americans, Hispanics, and Native Americans. There are also large groups of continental Europeans, Asians, Africans, and Middle-Easterners. Within these groups, diet and lifestyle vary due to cultural or religious customs passed down through the generations, and each group may have different attitudes toward food, exercise, weight, stress, and other lifestyle factors. Cultural factors provide the guiding principles by which we engage in society, and therefore in our health. Practitioners must work within those cultural constraints in order to engage the individual and prompt health changes.

23. WE ARE NOT SEPARATE FROM THE EARTH.   The Earth is our perfect environment. We have grown together, evolved together, and are nurtured together. From the clay of the Earth we were made, and it is from the minerals inherent in the soil that we receive our essential nourishment; we must intake minerals from outside food sources for existence. Every element, every mineral found in, on, or around the Earth can be found in our bodies. We were linked from the very beginning of creation.

When we defile the water, the land, the air, we only defile our place of residence. When we spill chemicals onto the Earth, we create degenerative disease in ourselves. When we damage the Earth, we damage our home. There is no spaceship coming to magically save us when we have trashed the Earth beyond its capacity to nourish us. When we damage and pollute the Earth, we are held closer to the ground, denser, thicker, and wetter. The glue that holds our cells together erodes; our bodies lose continuity and integrity. We devolve.

Geography holds a key to health improvement. With natural selection applications, our genes change very slowly over an evolutionary time frame. We are not too different from our ancestors from 500 or 2,000 years ago. Looking to the land of our ancestors may hold a key to our health, especially dietary requirements and disease tendencies.

For example, wheat was bred from grasses in the Fertile Crescent of the Middle East about 9,000 years ago, and spread into Europe, Britain, and the Far East about 5,000 years ago. In these areas, humans developed the enzymes and digestive actions to assimilate the nutrients from the grain. If your ancestors came from these areas, you may have the genetic capability to effectively digest traditionally prepared wheat products. On the other hand, if your ancestors came from Africa, the Indigenous New World, or Northern Europe, you may not have the genetic capability of digesting wheat. In which case, weight gain, bloating, and blood sugar swings may accompany digestive intolerance, or what we now call gluten sensitivity.

Another example: The ability to digest milk (lactose) is based upon an autosomal gene. If your ancestors came from Africa, Asia, the Mediterranean area, the indigenous populations of the New World or the Pacific area, there is a good chance you can't tolerate milk or other dairy products. On the other hand, if your ancestors are from northern Europe, eastern or central Europe, and parts of the Middle East or Somalia, there's a good chance you can continue to enjoy dairy through adulthood.

Take it back to the land, to the geography. What did your ancestors eat? You may have food sensitivities. How much sun exposure did they normally receive? This could affect your ability to make vitamin D. Take it back to the land—you won't be sorry.

Healthcare for All

These simple but basic tenets have guided folk healers and natural health practitioners for generations. Following these principles recognizes a holistic approach to healthcare grounded in traditional healing methods and value systems. It places the responsibility for wellness on the individual but denies healthcare to no one. It recognizes that we are all individual and that protocols should be also. It acknowledges the role of emotions, personality, and stress on health. And it acknowledges that we are made from the Earth and to the Earth we must look for our healing.

❧ THREE ❧

The Calling

*Every particular in nature, a leaf, a drop, a crystal, a
moment of time is related to the whole, and partakes of
the perfection of the whole.*

—*Ralph Waldo Emerson*

I WAS TOO YOUNG to pick cotton, so my mother let me run around the cotton field and play games with the other children of the field hands. My maternal grandfather, Papa Bright, was a sharecropper and planted cotton and corn to make his payments. Most of the field hands were family, so there were plenty of cousins to play hide-n-seek, to throw rocks and tell stories with, and to chase the little snippy bird, the killdeer, that builds its nest from the small sandstone pebbles that littered the field. All Southerners can tell a good story. It is part and parcel of our culture, and we learn early as children just how to tell the best tale.

There was a strip of grassy boundary land between the cotton field and the woods, and it was here that herbs and weeds of various sorts were found. It was here, among the sedge grasses that I loved to hide. If you lie flat in a field of sedge, there is nary a ripple in the flow of grass to mark your spot. I hid very well, and soon the other kids gave up trying to find me.

I was suddenly scared when I realized I was totally alone with the silence of the wind, the birds, and the insects. It was eerily quiet without human sound, and I was the only one of my kind in sight or hearing, no other humans. So I just lay in the sedge grass and stared at the sky, watching the white clouds move against the blue background. I listened to the sound of grasshoppers jumping among the grass stalks.

I could hear the birds talking among themselves in the nearby trees. And I could hear the wind ruffling the leaves of the trees and whispering through the needles of the pines.

I don't know how long I lay there, not moving, but I wasn't scared any longer. I had become part of the land, the cotton rows, the meadow, and the woods. We were the same, there was no separation. I fell asleep without a care in the world and didn't wake until Mama came looking for me. She was half angry that I had disappeared and no one knew where I was, and very angry that she had to leave her work to find me, but was glad I was alright. As we headed back to where she left her pick sack, I grabbed a ripe maypop (passionflower) and ate it as we walked.

This sort of peak experience with nature has happened over and over in my life. I can't remember a time when nature wasn't a part of my life—a friend, a teacher, a lover, an angry parent. Nature can be generous and abundant or cruel and hard. No one knows this better than a farmer or rancher.

It is this love of nature...this ability to merge into the landscape...that has sustained me whenever life has been uncertain. And it is this love of nature that quiets my soul and brings calm into my inner being even if I'm just sitting on the porch.

The Called

Traditionally, folk healers came to their professions by many different routes. One method, which I believe is still relevant, is the *calling*, an urge or drive that resonates so deeply within the psyche that to stray from the pathway could only bring internal conflict and pain. People who have a calling in an area generally have exceptional talent in that area.

Family history is also a strong predictor of embracing herbalism as a profession. Many sons or daughters go into medicine because their fathers were physicians. Likewise, many herbalists grow up learning from their mothers or fathers or grandmothers, and thus it is passed on.

Sometimes there are special circumstances around the birth of someone who has the talent for healing that is considered a sign. One of the most powerful examples is being *born with a caul* or veil over the face. The caul is part of the membrane, the amniotic sac, that covers the fetus in the womb and sometimes it sticks to the baby as it makes its way through the birth canal. This happens when the mother's water or amniotic sac does not break prior to the baby's birth.

Children born with the sac still intact have lower rates of neonatal infection as the sac protects the child immediately after birth. And for this reason, caul babies have a higher chance of surviving the first few weeks of life. Caul births are fairly rare these days, with fewer than one in 1,000 caul births. This is due to modern birthing methods such as breaking the water, generally for physician convenience, and the massive number of Caesarean section surgeries that are taking place. Premature babies, home-delivered babies, and quick labors most often yield caul babies.

Being born with a caul is considered a high sign that the child will be special, multitalented, and have extraordinary healing powers or the gift of second sight or prophecy. The child might also have a talent for music or art or generally have good luck. People born with the caul are thought to have the ability to see inside you, to know what is happening in your insides physically, emotionally, and spiritually. They are also thought to be able to see dead spirits.

In times past, the caul itself was considered a powerful healing and spiritual tool, and was dried and saved for future use. Bits of dried caul were often mixed into herbal formulas to heal the sick. And because it was considered protection from evil forces and demons, bits of dried caul were enclosed in lockets and worn around the neck or placed in small cases and carried in a pocket for protection. In previous centuries, the caul was bought and sold as a commodity on the open market. Sailors along the New England coast of North America believed that carrying a bit of caul would keep them from drowning.

Birth order is another indication of the gift of healing. Being born the seventh son or daughter is high sign of healing ability. And being born the seventh son or daughter of the seventh son or daughter, though rare, was believed to endow a person with extraordinary healing powers, the ability to see the future or prophesy, and the ability to stop the flow of blood. The mythology surrounding the seventh son is said to be related to the sacredness of the number seven in the Bible. With modern birth control methods giving rise to smaller families, being born the seventh child is becoming a rare event also.

Firstborn children have a special place in birth order because they inherit the gifts of the ancestors. The firstborn daughter of a firstborn daughter is said to inherit the accumulated healing power and wisdom of her mother, grandmother, and so on. Healing powers are considered strongest coming through the mother's line. The firstborn child after twins is endowed with special healing power that enables them to stop pain.

Children born after their father's death or children who have never seen their fathers are credited with being able to cure thrush by blowing into the baby's mouth, and may also have other special powers. According to tradition, these powers are God's compensation for taking away the father, whether he had died or skipped town.

Being born disfigured, handicapped, or with a prominent *birthmark* is a sign of special powers that can be used for either good or evil, and these folks must make a choice on how to use their gifts. Once a choice is made and a path chosen, it can not be recanted without the loss of their powers. In some Native American tribes, being born crippled, blind or deaf, or with other physical disabilities was seen as a sign, and these folks were generally trained as healers. On the practical side, this gave them a unique place in the tribe because their limited physical abilities prevented them from participating in the common hard physical labor that was necessary for survival, and from hunting or war games.

Being struck by *lightning* and surviving is another way to receive supernatural initiation. Thunderbolts from above cleanse and purge the body and leave behind power and magic. But it is also a sign that relationships are out of balance and a warning to return to emotional balance. Of course, the person struck by lightning may need to overcome its devastating effects on the nervous system if they survive.

In modern times, *wounded healers* are those who come to the healing profession because of their own life-threatening or chronic illness. Figuring out ways to improve their own health helps them transcend their illness and be transformed by the experience. This transformation propels them down a path of service and prompts a sharing of their experiences, knowledge, and healing journey with others. Wounded healers often believe they have been chosen as conduits for the healing power of God or that they are ill for a reason or because the illness is imparting a lesson. To take this action a step further, completely curing oneself from a serious illness provides a type of initiation which might also include moving into the dream world, seeing the ghosts of ancestors, or seeing visions.

Another way to receive the calling is through healing *dreams* or *visions*. Dr. Li, a Traditional Chinese doctor in my area, is the tenth generation of his family to be a healer, and so the tradition and knowledge run very deep within him. I once asked at what age he began his studies. Dr. Li answered, "As a small child I slept with my grandfather who passed on his knowledge in dreams."

Faith healers come to the healing professions as part of their spiritual life, having been called and empowered to do so by God. They heal by prayer, touch, or the laying on of hands. Their exceptional aptitude may include the ability to remove warts or stanch the flow of blood.

Faith healing also takes place within prayer groups, churches, and other spiritual environments. When I was growing up, our family depended upon the prayers of church folk and laying on of hands as a primary method of healing.

Fire-blowers or fire-talkers can take away the pain of burns or any pains that feel hot. This is done by blowing or sucking above, but not touching, the area of discomfort and then spitting out the energy of the pain onto the ground. A woman can teach a man how to fire blow and a man can teach a woman, but members of the same sex can't teach each other. This is also considered true of blood-stopping and wart-talking.

Blood-stoppers can stop the flow of blood from a bleeding nose or an open wound. The hand of the blood-stopper circles the head of the bleeding person three times while muttering a specific Bible verse. Ezekiel 16:6 is popular and so is the phrase, "Stop, blood, stop. Stop like God commanded the River of Jordan. Stop, blood, stop."

Wart-talkers can command a wart to disappear. There are several common techniques for this, such as rubbing a penny over the warts and throwing away the penny, rubbing a peeled potato over the warts and burying the potato, and by "charming" off the warts. My cousin Calvin was a wart-charmer and had quite a popular reputation based on his successes. He would place his hand over the warts and mutter a few secret phrases under his breath. He guaranteed the warts would disappear in three days and most often they did. I once asked Calvin how the charm worked. He replied, "My energy is stronger than the wart's energy." And that was that.

My Calling

As you can see, there are a lot of ways to be called to the healing professions. If you aren't born with any apparent special abilities, life's circumstances may still offer an unexpected route to the healing practices. I believe that everyone is born with some instinct for healthcare and healing, a certain perception of health priority that enables us to take normal care of ourselves and our families, if we pay attention to the inner voice. And then, some people are born with a special gift or talent for healing, just like some people are born with a talent for music or art.

Loving the land and everything growing upon it has given shape and strength to the foundation of who I am. That love has been compensation for some rough times, some poor times. I can't remember a time that being in the woods or reading, learning, seeking, finding, or sharing information about herbs and the body wasn't a priority in my life.

For some, the concept of Southern Folk Medicine as a complete and whole system, an American folk healing tradition, may be a new idea. I'm always amazed how few people realize its intricacies and completeness and its ease of use. One of my goals, part of my vision, is to help save Southern Folk Medicine, in all its forms, for future generations, and to help people help themselves. We can help ourselves, our families, our friends, our neighbors, and our clients with very simple home remedies and sound nutrition without running to the emergency room with every sneeze.

Folk herbalism, especially as was practiced in the South, is easy to understand and easy to use. You don't have to spend years learning a new system or familiarizing yourself with Chinese or Eastern Indian words or philosophies. The vocabulary is one that is already familiar, regardless of where you live. Its idioms are common and we have all heard our mothers and grandmothers use many of its phrases.

Folk herbalism in its purest form doesn't exist except in very isolated parts of the world. The last of the elders are passing away, and younger folks have lost interest in learning a natural approach to self-care. In addition, diverse cultural influences in this country continue to contribute simultaneously to the dilution and evolution of all folk medicines.

Growing up in North Alabama has truly been a gift. I remember standing in a cotton field as a child, feeling the earth rumble under my feet as booster rockets were being test fired at nearby NASA facilities. In my parent's life, they went from riding in wagons drawn by mules to witnessing space travel and the landing on the moon. Talk about a time warp! Sometimes I feel that I keep one foot in the past and one foot in the future—traditional knowledge anchors my foundation, and science propels me forward.

But I live in the present, as we all must do. And in the *now,* I believe that by codifying and sharing the information I learned as a child about Southern Folk Medicine and still practice, I can help people recover their health and reduce risk factors for chronic illness. I can help succeeding generations take personal responsibility for their health, and I can help save our folk medicines. If current environmental, sociopolitical, and healthcare trends continue, future generations are going to be even more health-challenged and in need of this healing information. Time is getting shorter and life is quite uncertain. Better to be prepared than not.

Like many other healers, I didn't come to my calling gently. I was born two weeks early after my mother slipped on some rocks when she and Daddy were fishing. It was a full moon on Friday the 13th of August. Because labor came on suddenly after the fall, I was born with a caul over my face. I was also born disfigured, with a cyst on my left breast which was surgically removed when I was six weeks old. My parents were told it was doubtful if I would ever be able to breast feed due to the scar tissue left behind, but I have breast fed all five of my children without problem. My mother was the oldest daughter in her family as I am. My love of herbs comes down through the paternal line of my family, through my Daddy's side, who counted themselves of Native American descent. If all this seems a bit metaphysical, well…yes, it is, and no, it ain't. It's just life, and I don't believe in random coincidences as a general rule.

After my initial folk education with various elders, I attended a local university and completed the requirements for a master's degree in health studies. I am continually teaching and learning and will never stop either as long as I have breath.

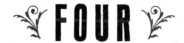

FOUR

Many Peoples, Many Traditions

The biggest difference between England and America is that England has history, while America has geography.

—Neil Gaiman

THE COTTON STALKS were sturdy and strong, around three to four feet; tall as a young girl. For the best yields, cotton needed to be spaced properly, just far enough apart to prevent crowding but close enough to fill the rows. It was chopped in the spring to remove broadleaf weeds that might choke out the cotton, and it was during this time that the cotton was also thinned. As a young girl, I became expert at thinning a row, eyeing the number of very small cotton plants that needed removing while leaving the strongest plants for best yields. All across the cotton field, you could hear the sound of many hoe blades clipping into the earth and striking against the small pebbles in the soil—chop, chop, chopping down into the dirt as folks moved along a row. That's why it was called chopping cotton. It was a distinct sound, and even now I can hear that sound-memory as I write.

But today was a nice fall day and cotton-picking time. I was small for my age, skinny and not very strong. I would gather handfuls of cotton and put in Mama's pick sack. When I was older and stronger, I was given a small pick sack, half the size of an adult one, and put on the row next to Mama to work along. I was never much good at picking and would fall behind the adult pickers. The days were long and hot, and the cotton rows were longer yet, and my attention easily wandered. Cotton was paid by the pound and I could work and struggle all day and barely pick 25 cents worth of the fluffy stuff.

A cotton stalk can grow up to five feet tall. I'm always amused in movies when they show cotton stalks about twelve inches tall. Yes, picking cotton is back-breaking work, but that is ridiculous. That little short cotton of the movies is perfect for the mechanical cotton picker and is the cotton planted today. That was not the cotton of my youth. On this day, the stalks were almost as tall as me and just right for a little girl to stand upon the bottom two branches and balance, for just a tiny fraction of a second before it bent. It was almost impossible to break a cotton stalk. This cousin of the hemp plant has fibrous stalks that defied the strongest hands and sharpest knives. The stalk would bend rather than break. And so the cotton stalk and I floated to the ground together before Mama yelled at me to "Behave." But I was a magician escaping from an evil sorcerer who wanted my powers. I floated slowly to the ground upon a winged stallion and escaped his evil clutches. "Behave, I said." Mama's voice once again cut through the fantasy, bringing me back to the cotton field. She was pulling ahead in the row and so I hurried to catch up.

It was one of those Alabama autumn mornings—clean and crisp with just a of bite of chill in the air. The smell of leaf mold and wood smoke filled my nostrils. It would be hot by the afternoon, but the morning was divine. This was perfect cotton-picking weather, and here my mama's family was spending their days. Papa Bright was a sharecropper and worked Mrs. Cranford's land. She was a good woman, a widow woman, whose husband had died when she was fairly young and left her with some land and a young son. Mrs. Cranford wasn't a demanding woman nor a greedy one, and was a friend to the family even after Papa Bright retired.

The old farmhouse where my grandparents lived didn't have indoor plumbing, but neither did ours nor any other members of the family. It did boast a well across the road from the house and another on the back porch. Many a time Papa Bright would draw a bucket of water and put it on the front porch with a dipper for us kids to drink during the day while the grownups worked the fields.

Because Papa Bright was a hunter, there was often a hide tacked to the wall of the house curing in the shade of the porch. It was basically a shotgun house with another section added onto the west side making an L-shape. The outhouse was in the backyard, complete with various catalogues including the *Sears Catalogue* and the *Farm Journal Magazine*. Papa Bright had never learned to read but could do his numbers extremely well and would flip through the farming magazine looking at the photos, and when he was done, the magazine became toilet paper.

The four-room house was built on stacked rocks of various sizes and shapes that precariously formed pillars under it, at the corners, and at various points along the outside walls. The stones were dry-stacked, without the use of mortar, and no two stones were the same size or shape. There were several reasons for this architectural design. The odd-sized and -shaped stone pillar design was believed to keep out termites, and I can't say this isn't true. Many of these old houses have been abandoned across the South for years and years and are still solid and standing, without a hint of termite damage.

Because the foundation was open, a cool breeze circulated under the house, cooling off the occupants in a time before air conditioning. Under the house, the dogs wallowed out depressions in the sandy soil, staying cool in the summer and warm in the winter. The open foundation plan also eliminated any moisture problems under the house. The air was always circulating, and therefore moisture never built. This was a unique style that combined elements of European, African, and Native American building techniques—one that was perfectly suited to the climate of the South and the building materials at hand.

There were two chimneys in the house. The main heating came from a rock-and-mortar chimney on the east side to accommodate a small coal fireplace. Instead of using the inefficient fireplace, my grandparents connected a coal-burning stove to the chimney, which furnished better heat to the surrounding rooms than a small fireplace could ever do. This was the main room of the house and in true old-fashioned style, it was both the living room and the main bedroom, with a four-poster bed along one wall and a couch along the other. Papa Bright's easy chair was firmly in place next to the stove and by a window. Here he spent many a winter hour smoking his home-rolled cigarettes or pipe, thinking and staring out the window—waiting once again for planting time.

The other chimney was in the kitchen. It was little more than a rock-and-mortar tunnel through the roof and to vent the wood-burning kitchen stove. On this stove, Mama Bright prepared all family meals, including the meals for the field hands. In those days, Papa Bright believed that if a man or woman worked your fields, were your hands, then you were obliged to pay them and furnish them with a noonday meal. Mama Bright prepared dinner, modernly called lunch, on the wood stove. It was a plain but hearty meal with meat, beans, potatoes, cornbread, some type of vegetables from the garden, and a dessert such as sweet potato pie or cobbler, with coffee for the adults and fresh milk for the children. The field hands ate first, and the leftover food was given to us children. This wasn't a cruel gesture; it was practical. The people who had to bend their backs and pull the heavy pick sacks needed all the energy available, so they ate first.

On this autumn day, everyone who was going to be picking cotton met at the farmhouse to caravan to the field. I climbed into the back of Papa Bright's pickup truck along with the cousins. The sideboards were built extra tall, and it was here that the pick sacks were emptied after they were weighed. Mama followed in the car so when the day was done, we could head straight home without going back to the farm. On this day, there was cotton in the back of the truck left from the previous afternoon's pickings. Once the cotton reached the top of the sideboards, Papa Bright would go to the cotton gin, where it would be weighed and then sucked out the back of the pickup truck with the strongest vacuum imaginable. I loved going to the gin with him and watching this.

Our empty pick sacks were stretched out over the cotton and formed a blanket over the softness as we bounced along the edge of the cotton field and over terraced rows, holding onto the sideboards or each other to keep from bouncing about or out. It was just family in the back of the truck. Any child too young to either help pick or run around the cotton field unattended was left with Mama Bright.

Papa seldom hired extra field hands. He was just too poor and there wasn't enough cotton picked to pay those not in the family, but on occasion, when the yield was extra good or speed of harvest was important, he hired extra help. This was one of those times. The cotton had to be picked by the end of the week.

We didn't often see black people where we lived; there had never been any plantations in the area because it was mountaintop land. But cotton was king and if there was an acre of flat land, then cotton was planted. Papa Bright worked fields all over the mountain because of this—5 acres here and 40 acres there, and so on. The majority of the time, the field hands were white.

Today was different—a black man was going to pick with us. I thought he must have come a long, long way to pick cotton. The only other time I had ever seen a black man was on Papa Bright's front porch. Three black men had stopped one rainy afternoon to buy some rabbits Papa Bright had killed when hunting. All us cousins had peeped through the window in total curiosity. Our Uncle had told us that black men liked to cut off the ears of little white girls and put them in their stew. And then he had looked straight at me and said they especially liked little red-headed girl's ears the best and I should be extra careful. I remembered his words as I stood on the edge of the cotton field and stared at the new field hand, both simultaneously intrigued and fearful.

Of course, I didn't stop to think that my uncle himself also threatened to cut off our ears every time we got in his way or messed with his dogs. He would pull out his pocket knife and start cleaning his fingernails. We would know right then that we were in trouble and would run for our lives. On one occasion, a cousin had lost a bolt from the motor he was rebuilding, and Uncle had actually chased us around and around the house, knife drawn. We had all run and squealed and finally made our escape into the cornfield next to the house, but none of us ever bothered his tools again.

As the morning wore away, I caught myself edging closer and closer to the black man, and when Papa Bright called for the morning weigh-in, I found myself wandering through the plants that grow in the border between the woods and field. The weigh-in was held four times a day—mid-morning, dinner, mid-afternoon, and the close of the day. The cotton was weighed on the scales that hung on an extended sideboard off the back of the truck. Weigh-in was also the time to rest, get some water, and have a snack. Folks chatted and gossiped a bit during the weigh-in, but everyone got quiet when their sack was being weighed. They wanted to know how much they were earning because cotton was paid by the pound. And there was always a bit of competition to see who had picked the most.

Me, I enjoyed just running around the fields, making crowns out of dried cotton bolls, looking at the plants, and finding pretty sandstone pebbles. Between the woods and the field was a wide strip of grassland that was full of plants. I wandered among the plants picking goldenrod, maypop, and aster during the weigh-in. "Those purple flowers are good for fever," said the black man motioning to the asters. "I know," I replied rather shyly, barely whispering the words. "What about those yellow ones?" he asked. I shrugged a "don't know." "Those are good for the kidneys and passing water," he said. I looked at the goldenrod with new respect and continued my wandering. "These are good to eat," I said pointing to the passionflower. "And them leaves will help you sleep," he added. And then it was time to get back to working the fields. I followed along after him off and on for the rest of the day, sometimes asking questions and sometimes in silence. He let me sit on the end of his pick-sack and scooted me along until it got too full and heavy and he needed to pack the cotton down into the space where I had been sitting. Anyone who'd let me do that was definitely my friend.

As we were heading home at the end of the day, Mama backed the car off a terrace row. The back wheels were barely touching the Earth and the car just couldn't get any traction. We just sort of hung there, not going anywhere. Luckily, my friend hadn't left yet and so put his already tired back and shoulders into moving the car as Mama pressed the gas. I was on my knees in the backseat peering out the rearview window as the wheels caught and we drove away. I waved goodbye and he waved to me, and I never saw him again. Cotton-picking was done.

Many years have passed since those cotton field days. I like to think that just as Southern Folk Medicine has its roots in many cultures, so does our family, which is now mixed with many cultures and many colors…all the richer for the diversity.

Many Peoples, Many Traditions

The origins of Southern Folk Medicine cannot be pinned to a specific time or place. As an oral tradition, which has been passed from generation to generation, its origins were never truly documented. It evolved as the need arose, the way any folk medicine is wont to do. As a result, referenced material is very scarce and based on anecdotal stories, diaries, and interviews of practitioners and common folk. What little documentation that does exist is more about its practices and principles and its use of plant remedies rather than its origins.

The South didn't boast a unified culture until the Civil War. The origins of what is now the Southern states were very different from those of the Northeast United States. For example, the Carolinas and Georgia were settled and controlled by the English, and Georgia was originally settled by debtors and criminals as one of the thirteen original colonies. Spain maintained control of Florida until the early 1800s when it was absorbed into the United States. During the seventeenth and eighteenth centuries, control of the region that later became

Alabama, Mississippi, parts of Tennessee, Arkansas, and Louisiana went back and forth between Spain and France. Parts of Tennessee and Kentucky had first been under French control but later shifted to the British.

Documentation of Southern Folk Medicine principles and practices can be found in several broad categories of sources that can be easily accessed by the general public. Of great importance are books, diaries, and journals written by explorers, invaders, and settlers to the New World. Especially helpful are the journals written by physicians and botanists who accompanied Spanish explorers here. Books and newspaper articles written during and immediately after the American Civil War provide a wealth of information by physicians, pharmacists, herbalists, and housewives who had no choice but to use herbal medicine as primary care because the South was in a blockade by land and sea, and processed medicines were only available as trade contraband in an illegal market.

After the Civil War, books and articles written by individuals, medical botanists, and pre-1900 physicians continued to document the use of Southern Folk Medicine, especially among poor blacks and whites. Interviews conducted during the Great Depression by the Folklore Project and the American Slave Narratives project of the Federal Writers' Project of the Works Progress Administration, which are housed in the Library of Congress, provide information about the use of botanicals for healing. And finally, sociological studies and interviews conducted by universities and private foundations on folkways in America from the 1970s to the 1980s provide another layer of information. While documentation is scarce, oral tradition remained rich until the 1980s, when conventional medicine became more accessible due to an increase in the number of physicians in the South and some access to health insurance. However, those living in poverty or those disillusioned with modern medicine continue to use herbal and home remedies as their primary medical care today.

It is not the focus of this book to dig through historical documents and reference each and every bit of information that graces these pages. Most of what I write about is based on oral tradition and hasn't left a footprint. My intention is to document and codify the folk medicine that I was taught through oral tradition, that was handed down, so it isn't lost forever. It is important that the tradition is saved.

Southern and Appalachian Folk Medicine is a melding, a blending of several healing modalities from several cultures that came together to create something unique. Each culture contributed vital knowledge and practices to the beginnings of a new healthcare framework for a New World. Upon this fertile land, European conventional medicine, influenced by Greek or humoral medicine, Native American plant use, African spiritual practices, and Irish folk medicine practices, combined to form Southern and Appalachian Folk Medicine.

Let's explore the beginnings of a unique folk system.

Early Explorations

The beginnings of American history and folk medicine didn't originate with Plymouth Rock, but in the woodlands and swamps of the American South. By the time the English landed at Plymouth Rock, the South had been explored and settled for almost 100 years, and the origins of our traditional folk medicine had been set. Because of this, many people in the South, including me, carry Spanish blood whether they know it or not.

The primary goals of Spanish exploration and invasion of the New World were simple and basic: accumulate riches, especially gold; develop a source of slaves for the building of the Spanish empire; and find the shortcut to China to break the monopoly on spices held by the Ottoman Empire. The conversion of the indigenous peoples of the New World to Christianity was a corollary goal of the expedition; therefore, Spanish priests arrived with the explorers. The combination of intense, almost obsessive, Christian religious beliefs with humoral medicine was unrestrained during this time in Europe. It *was* the medicine of Europe. In the New World, coupled with Native American knowledge of plant use, this combination forms the unmistakable foundations of Southern Folk Medicine.

In the early 1500s, under the hot Southern sun, the first adventurers to the New World, Spanish explorers and their Moorish slaves, made their way through humid forests in search of the ever-elusive shortcut to China and the procurement of mythical treasures of gold, silver, and gems said to be hidden by the natives. The expeditions included healers and physicians who practiced humoral medicine based on the works of Galen and Avicenna, and who knew how to fight as well as care for the wounded. Some expeditions also brought botanists and naturalists to draw and describe the exotic plant and animal life of the New World, as well as historians to chronicle the exploits and adventures of the expeditions, especially to extol the leaders.

In 1526, Lucas Vasquez de Ayllon led 600 Spanish colonists and their Northern African slaves to settle on a South Carolina bay, ninety-four years before the Pilgrims founded Plymouth (1620). Disease and hunger reduced the vitality, strength, and, ultimately, the number of Spanish, and provided an easy opportunity for their African slaves to revolt and flee into the surrounding land where they took up residence with local Native Americans, the first peoples of the New World. Disease ravaged the remaining Spanish colonists who couldn't survive without slaves to help with hard labor. The colony soon disbanded and the survivors returned to Spain, leaving the runaway slaves to either die in the wilderness or be assimilated into Native American tribes. This pattern was to be repeated several times over the course of colonization: Europeans such as the Spanish arrived with their Northern African slaves, and the slaves ran off to join the Native Americans.

St. Augustine in Florida represents the first permanent settlement in the New World. The fort of St. Augustine was built forty-two years before the English settled Jamestown and fifty-five years before the Pilgrims landed at Plymouth Rock. In 1565, Admiral Don Pedro Menendez de Aviles, and his men and slaves, took over and fortified an Indian village, claiming the land for Spain. Named for the patron saint of theologians and printers, and on whose birthday the Spanish fleet landed, the settlement represented an attempt to outflank the French who had established a colony on the St. Johns River and were threatening Spanish interests. But Menendez, one of Spain's most brilliant generals, quickly rid the land of the French and claimed it for Spain. Luckily, a timely hurricane aided his endeavors by eliminating the French fleet.

Fairly soon, Spain controlled most of what was to become the United States, as well as Central and South America and the Caribbean. Colonies and settlements were established in the future states of North Carolina, South Carolina, Florida and Louisiana, New Mexico, California, and Arizona. The results of these encounters for Native Americans were disastrous, as European diseases decimated their populations and wiped out whole villages.

French colonization in the South was generally restricted to the Gulf area and along the Mississippi River. Like the Spanish, the French also brought slaves from western Africa, mostly from Senegal, to support their efforts at colonization in the New World. The city of Mobile, Alabama, the first planned city in the United States, with streets and boulevards, was designed by the French.

We can see that by the early 1500s, the first interactions in the New World occurred between the Spanish, their Moorish slaves, and the Native Americans. Information exchange was already taking place, especially that relating to foods and healing knowledge.

The European humoral system of medicine became integrated with Native American uses of plants rather quickly, due to survival issues. For this reason, Southern Folk Medicine has much in common with the post-Columbian folk medicines of Mexico, parts of Central and South America, and especially the Caribbean. We share the same origins. Adding the layer of Irish folk medicine really increases the similarities between Caribbean Folk Medicine and Southern Folk Medicine.

De Soto and His Legacy

In 1538, Hernando de Soto arrived in Cuba with his wife, several priests, a few slaves, and a large entourage. For the next year, as governor of Cuba, de Soto finalized his preparations for the exploration of the American continent. With a mission from the King of Spain to find a route between the Atlantic and Pacific oceans, de Soto began recruiting men and preparing supplies for an extended exploration. De Soto's success in Peru in 1532, with Pizarro, had earned him a reputation as a hero of conquest in Spain. For this reason, many men were willing to join the potentially profitable exploration and conquest of the new lands.

Expecting to find gold, silver, and precious stones to compensate their travels, the band of more than 600 soldiers were very disappointed and surprised to find the natives of North America did not hold these objects to be valuable, as the Incas did. Nor were the Native Americans as docile as expected; the Spanish found no submission of them as they had the Incas. Even the Native women would take up bow and arrow when the Native men fell to de Soto's rampages.

De Soto chose to follow the same ill-fated route through Florida as a previous explorer, Narvaez, who also met the Apalachee tribe while searching for gold and the ever-elusive shortcut to China. According to the journal of the Gentleman of Elvas, a Portuguese member of the de Soto expedition and author of *The De Soto Chronicles,* "As soon as they reached Cale, the governor ordered all the maize which was ripe in the field to be taken, which was enough for three months. When they were gathering this, the Indians killed three Christians, and one of two Indians who were captured told the governor that seven days' journey farther on was a very large province with maize in abundance, called Apalache." De Soto set off for this land, wreaking havoc and carnage along the way and taking Indian slaves to ground the maize with mortar and bake it into flat pieces on earthen vessels set onto the fire. De Soto continued his journey to Apalache looking for maize, gold, and other riches.

The Gentleman of Elvas chronicles de Soto's march up through Florida and Georgia, through the lower Carolinas, and back down through Tennessee, Alabama, and the Midwestern states. The chronicler did note of the Native diet: "their ordinary food is maize, in place of bread, and their viands are beans and calabashes....Their drink is clear water, just as nature gives it to them, without the admixture of anything else. The meat and the fish they eat must be very well dressed and cooked, and the fruit very ripe. They will never eat it green or half-ripe and laugh at the Castilians for eating green fruit."

The De Soto Chronicles tell very little about the everyday lives of the natives. Rather, the book is focused upon the feats and campaigns of an army razing the land. One particular battle, however, the Battle of Mauvila, stands out from other battle descriptions due to the particular type of medicine the Spaniards used after a particularly bloody battle, one where all soldiers had some type of wound and many had five or ten. The chronicler writes that during the battle, all provisions, including the medicines, had been consumed by fire, leaving the surgeon with no medicines to treat so many wounded. All food, shelter, and the trappings of communion had also burned. The chronicler writes: "They made roofs from the arbors to fasten to the walls that were left standing. Others busied themselves in cutting open the dead Indians and taking the fat to use as ointment and oil in treating wounds." Human fat was used in place of the olive oil normally the surgeon would have used to dress wounds but which had perished in the fire.

The de Soto troop never experienced firsthand living with the natives as had Cabeza, a Spaniard who explored Texas, the West, and Mexico. Instead de Soto viewed the land as an adversary, one to be conquered and so too the very people who lived upon it. Many Spaniards died from lack of salt, and only in desperation did they try the Native remedy. The account from the chronicler: "Having passed some days without it [salt], they felt the lack of it greatly, and some whose constitutions required more than others died for the need of it in a most extraordinary manner." A fever developed, followed by a terrible stench from the body, which lasted for several days until the Spaniard came strongly upon them and death followed. The chronicler writes that "their bellies were as green as grass from the breast down."

After several deaths, some of the remaining soldiers "made use of the remedy the Indians [slaves] prepared to save and help themselves in that necessity. This was that they burned a certain herb they knew about and made lye with the ashes. They dipped what they ate in it as if it were a sauce and with this they saved themselves from rotting away and dying, like the Spaniards." Some high-ranking Spaniards refused the remedy, regarding it as "unbecoming to their rank," and died for their stupidity and pride. More than sixty Spaniards died in the year of no salt. The salt famine ended when they discovered brackish water with blue sand. Recognizing this as saltpeter, they decided it could be made into powder for their weapons. After straining the blue sand through water, it was brought to a boil and converted into a yellowish salt. Several of the soldiers "ate it by itself in mouthfuls, as if it were sugar." In a few days, these men died of dropsy (edema).

I've often wondered if the lack of apparent and readily accessible salt which the Spanish found in the New World influenced the prominent role that salt plays in the foundation of Southern Folk Medicine. In Southern Folk Medicine, salt (sodium) is connected to the element of water.

The De Soto Chronicles provides a wealth of information about the interactions of the Spanish and the Native Americans, including food and herb use. *The Chronicles* specifically mention oaks, walnuts, sweetgum, pines, corn, beans, prickly pears, squashes, saw palmetto, mulberries, sarsaparilla, sumac, wild olives, and various herbs and roots.

De Soto died from fever and was buried in the Mississippi River. He explored parts of the Appalachian Mountains and, according to some historians, named them after the Apalachee Indian tribe of northern Florida. His explorations continued through the South and Midwest, and he is credited as being the first European to see the Mississippi River. De Soto's brutality toward the Native populations is well-chronicled. Enough said.

New World Plant Influences

For the Europeans, finding new medicines required travel outside of Europe, and some Spanish physicians and botanists believed that the New World offered a unique supply. In 1569, Nicolas Monardes, a Spanish physician and botanist, published *Medical Study of the Products Imported from our West Indian Possessions,* which contained descriptions of seventy-five plants and their medicinal uses. Interestingly, the genus Monarda was named after him. His book included the first written therapeutic benefits of such common herbs as tobacco, which Monardes believed to be an antidote to poisons, and sassafras, which was believed could cure syphilis. Monardes also believed that tobacco was a panacea for most any health issue including head colds, stomach problems, wounds, old sores, women's health issues, and cancer.

In addition to the slew of physical ailments healed by tobacco, Monardes also recorded spiritual uses of the plant: "One of the marvels of this Herb, and that which does bring most admiration, is, the manner how the priests of the Indies did use of it.… " Monardes also recorded the use of tobacco by the average person to improve energy, create relaxation, and calm weariness—and, as a recreational drug, "In like sort the rest of the Indians for their pastime, do take the smoke of the Tobacco, for to make them selves drunk withal, and to see the visions, and things that do represent to them, wherein they do delight."

The following passage illustrates an example how explorers, settlers, and slaves learned the use of local herbs from the Native populations. Monardes also writes, "The black people that have gone from these parts to the Indies, has taken the same manner and use of the Tobacco, that the Indians have, for when they see themselves weary, they take it at the nose, and mouth, and it does happen unto them, as unto our Indians, lying as though they were dead three or four hours: and after they do remain lightened, without any weariness, for to labor again.… "

While we might think of tobacco as being a purely North American herb, with over sixty species, some species of Nicotiana grew from Canada to the tip of South America. This is an herb of the *Americas* and from here spread to the rest of the world. *Nicotiana tabacum* is a tall, broad-leaf, attractive plant which Native Americans were already cultivating when Columbus arrived. Plant geneticists believe that the center of origin for the tobacco plant was the Andes, and that it later spread to all part of the Americas. *Nicotiana rustica,* or wild tobacco, is smaller, less showy, and has much larger amounts of the alkaloid nicotine. This plant was more often used in healing ceremonies, spiritual rituals, and as a poison. Native Americans partook of tobacco in pipes, as tea, in powder as snuff, and in cigars. All methods of application are still in use today. I've often wondered what ancient Native Americans would have thought about the way tobacco has been corrupted and misused.

Monardes also wrote about the magic of sassafras. He believed sassafras was a gift from God for the treatment of venereal diseases, especially syphilis. It could also treat the many fevers of unknown origin and seasoning diseases that Spanish explorers and settlers often experienced in the New World. As Donald Beecher writes, "Monardes believed in the power of sassafras to the point where he carried a piece of the wood on his person to protect himself from the contagions and pestilences he encountered as a practicing doctor—for which singular virtue he praised God for this marvelous plant." John Frampton translated Monardes's work into English in 1577, with the title *Joyful News Out of the New Found World.*

In addition to documentation of the uses of sassafras by Monardes, Jacques Cartier also documented its use in 1535. Brian A. Honen, MPH, writes "England was so desperate for this new valuable medicine that Sir Walter Raleigh helped establish during the late 1580s, 'great woods of Sassafras' were noted to be in the vicinity in 1585." Because sassafras was believed to cure syphilis, by 1620, it became the first overharvested plant of the New World.

The Old World, Europe, was so desperate for any new medicine that, according to Stefanie Gänger in her 2015 paper "World Trade in Medicinal Plants from Spanish America, 1717–1815," "by the eighteenth century, 'foreign' plant-based remedies were passed on to the urban and rural poor [in Spain] by religious orders, private charity or, from the late eighteenth century, increasingly systematic medical relief programmes." Fortunately, the Spanish were quite adept at documenting the Indigenous peoples of the New World as well as plants and animals found in the land.

Spain wasn't the only country adopting New World plants into their official pharmacopeias. English historians, botanists, and illustrators were also busy, though Spain had a head start. Virgil J. Vogel, in *American Indian Medicine,* writes that the "most celebrated plant remedy to reach the world by way of the Carolinas was the Indian pinkroot (Spigelia marilandica L.), a Cherokee remedy for worms, which was adopted into the London, Dublin, and Edinburg pharmacopeias...." Pinkroot was considered safe for children if given with a mild laxative and was greatly in demand in Europe, which led to its overharvesting and is still considered endangered today.

Other plants of the New World which became economically and medically important in Europe included American ginseng, sweetgum, sarsaparilla, cayenne, dogwood, Seneca snakeroot, pleurisy root, also known as butterfly weed, yucca, evening primrose, white oak, white pine, elderberry, raspberry, and cedar berries. Many of these new and intriguing plant-based medicines made their way from Europe to India, Africa, and China.

As an aside, new foods also made their way from the New World to Europe. It is not the scope of this book to discuss New World foods in detail; however, it does bear a mention. Popular and important foods and spices from the New World include potatoes, sweet potatoes, peanuts, cayenne, pineapple, avocado, mango, papaya, allspice, cocoa, tomatoes, coca leaf, corn, beans, squashes, amaranth, quinoa, yacon, guarana, vanilla, and soursop. From the North American New World, Europe also received pecans, black walnuts, persimmons, blueberries and huckleberries, cranberries, prickly pears, sunflowers, pumpkins, strawberries, paw paws, American chestnuts, and maple syrup.

It also bears mentioning that another plant of New World origin—cotton—later became the economic cornerstone of the Southern United States. Upland cotton or *Gossypium hirsutism,* native to Central America, Mexico, the Caribbean, and southern Florida became so economically important that it now comprises 90 percent of the cotton grown worldwide. A discussion of cotton would be a whole other book, but the demand for it played an important role in the culture of the South and my childhood.

One last point to consider: Plants have been exchanged across the world since the beginning of trade among peoples. Plants from the New World scattered across Europe, India, and the Far East, while plants from these same areas found homes in the New World. Wherever people migrate, their plants tend to migrate with them. In addition, governments that subsidized exploration to the New World also expected a return on their investment. Plants useful as medicine or food or as garden ornamentals became part of that investment return and were broadly traded.

The Southern United States is one of the most diverse regions of the country. I'm fortunate to live in Alabama, which alone has more than 4,533 species of plants and ranks fifth in the nation for overall biodiversity, fourth in the nation for exceptional biodiversity, and number two in the nation for species extinction risk. Think of all the potential medicine that our ancestors accessed and that we are ignoring today! I do worry that climate change and the loss of habitat due to urbanization and deforestation will greatly increase the extinction of many species that are potential remedies and medicines. What if the cure for cancer was in the deep Alabama forests? How will we know unless we protect and investigate?

Naturalists today bemoan the number of invasive plant species from Europe and Asia that have found new homes in this country such as privet, kudzu, camphor tree, tree of heaven, fence rose, wisteria, Japanese knotweed, mimosa, sweet autumn, and purple loosetrife. But this cuts both ways. While European privet was invading the South, black locust (Robinia pseudoacacia) from the South was invading Britain and parts of Europe and Africa.

A Very, Very Brief History of Humoral Medicine

In addition to other Old World cultural elements, Spanish physicians and soldiers brought the conventional medicine of Europe to the New World. Its basis was in Greek or humoral medicine (hereafter known as humoral medicine), and embodied various theories and practices that evolved over centuries in the Mediterranean region. Later, known as Galenic medicine, Greek medicine spread across Europe, continuing to evolve along the way and taking on regional and cultural variations. Galenic medicine was used by European and Spanish physicians and influenced Western conventional medicine until the nineteenth century.

Like many folk medicines, humoral medicine was not initially a uniform system, but was drawn from the region's diverse areas, climates, and spiritual belief systems. Most likely the Greek humoral system was influenced somewhat by ancient Egypt, whose physicians were considered the finest in the area.

The Egyptians also documented their herbal and medical practices. The Kahoun Papyrus dates from 1825 BCE and includes sections on herbs, surgery, and diagnostics. The Ebers Papyrus, a 110-page herbal text that dates to 1550 BCE, was copied from earlier texts and offers a wealth of information. The ancient Egyptians believed that the heart was the organ most responsible for good health and the center of fluid movement around the body. Already you can see the beginnings of the humoral system in the ancient writings.

The Ebers Papyrus accurately describes such conditions as angina pectoris, aneurysm, and hernia. It discusses how to examine all the body fluids, including blood, mucus, urine, perspiration, tears, and feces. Also noted were the use of nutrition for health, the limbs, color of skin and face, quality of light in the eyes, and the smell of sweat, breath, and the body fluids. Most important to the examination was the taking of the pulse and the temperature of various parts of the body. This was, to say the least, a complete and thorough physical examination based on observational signs and the symptoms reported by the patient, a lost art in our modern approach to medicine where physical assessment skills are often left to machines and technology.

Ancient Egyptians believed that some illness was the result of angering the Gods. However, the physicians also used a theory based on the channels that farmers dug for irrigation. The heart was the center of forty-six channels that ran through the body. If any of the channels became blocked, illness could occur. Herbs, movement, and spiritual practices were designed to unblock the channels or appease the gods and allow the fluids to move freely. For example, mental illness was believed to be the result of blocked channels and angering the gods.

Many of the herbal remedies used by ancient Egyptians are still in use today for the same health issues or disorders. For example, garlic was used for asthma, pneumonia, and other bronchopulmonary complaints. We now know that when the sulfur compounds in garlic are metabolized, there is a concentrate of the compounds in the lungs, sweat, and urine. That's why garlic lovers have garlic breath and can stop a vampire at twenty-five paces. Garlic was used for sore throat and earache, both modern herbal uses also. Castor oil was used as a laxative, cedar oil as an antiseptic, and willow for pain reduction. All of these are still in use. This supports the concept in folk medicine that if a remedy works, it continues in use. If a remedy doesn't work, it drops out of the repertoire.

In ancient Greece, humoral medicine had its roots in the Cult of Asclepius, who was considered the God of Medicine. Asclepius was the son of the god Apollo and the mortal Coronas, but was raised by the centaur Chiron, who taught Asclepius the healing arts. It is said that Chiron was the first teacher of medicine and knew all the uses of the plants. In addition to skill in herbal crafts, Chiron also taught healers to use prayer, incantations, ointments, and surgery for healing.

Asclepius carried a staff with a serpent intertwined around it (the symbol of modern medicine) and became so good at healing that he could revive the dead. Raising the dead was a crime against the natural order and brought Asclepius to the attention of Mount Olympus. Zeus, fearing that the land would become overpopulated, killed Asclepius with a thunderbolt and carried him to Mount Olympus to become a god. Asclepius, God of Medicine, married Epione, Goddess of Soothing Pain, and had four daughters, all of whom worked in the healing arts. Hygeia was the Goddess of Good Health; Panacea, the Goddess of Curatives and Medicines; Aceso, the Goddess of Healing and Curing; and Iaso, the Goddess of Remedies and Modes of Healing. A young man, Telesphoros, the God of Convalescence, is often seen with Asclepius, but the relationship between the two is unclear.

The Cult of Asclepius began about the sixth century BCE with temples built around Greece and later Rome. The temples were a cross between a spa, a hospital, and a religious site where the sick could go for healing. While the Cult of Asclepius created priests, it also gave birth to a family of physicians who claimed direct descendance from Asclepius and are considered the true source of Greek medicine.

However, it was Hippocrates (460–370 BCE) and his students who first defined and wrote about humoral medicine in a functional and scientific manner. They were also the first physicians to recognize that illness had a natural cause, in contrast to the more superstitions views of the time, which related the cause of illness to supernatural influences.

Hippocrates's contributions to medicine stand to this day. In addition to being the first to place and order healing knowledge into a scientific system, Hippocrates and his students were the first to separate magic from medicine and to make medicine a profession. Hippocrates was a teacher and the founder of a school of medicine that flourished for several hundred years and influenced conventional medicine for over 2,000 years. Hippocrates's *Corpus* is a collection of work that spans the fifth and fourth centuries BCE and discusses a wide range of topics such as diseases of women, epidemics, and surgery. Much of Hippocrates's writings are still available today.

Galen (129–c. 200 AD) further refined and expanded the basic concepts of Hippocrates's humoral system. His views on medicine were developed using both empiricism and observation, believing that experience was the best teacher, but that theoretical knowledge also held a place in the study and application of medicine.

He began his early studies in the temples of Asclepius but later moved to Rome and became a physician at the Roman court. Galen believed that disease was caused by an imbalance in the humors, but unlike Hippocrates who believed the humors were imbalanced over the entire body, Galen believed the humors could become imbalanced within an organ or localized area as well. He believed in experimentation to increase knowledge, in dissection, and in the Vital Spirit. He discovered veins, arteries, and the movement of blood around the body and felt the pulse as a form of diagnosis. Galen categorized herbs according to their energetic properties: heating, cooling, moistening, or drying. Much of his work is still applicable today.

Galen's influence on the humoral model crafted early folk medicine into university-worthy teaching material. This is one of the reasons the Greek humoral system became known as Galenic medicine.

Galenic medicine lost prominence as physicians began to view the body as a mechanical entity rather than spiritual one. But this was a slow process and occurred over time. Galen's medicine continued to influence the view of the body even after the discovery of the germ theory. In addition to his own works and writings, Galen also offered commentaries on Hippocrates's writing. About a third of Galen's writings survive today; that's about three million words. His writings influenced both Western and Islamic medicines.

Other influential physicians and writers of the humoral system include Avicenna, an Arab philosopher, physician, and brilliant medical scholar who contributed the idea that disease could be contagious. Like Hippocrates, Avicenna thought that disease could be distributed by water or land. He believed that psychology influenced health and believed in the mind/body connection. This prodigy wrote the *Canon of Medicine* at a young age, which is still in print today.

While there were many other influential physicians, herbalists, and healers of Galenic medicine, the works of these three formed the foundation of humoral healing knowledge. Other authors I also suggest include Dioscorides (40–90), Hildegard of Bingen (1098–1179), Maimonides (1135–1204), Paracelsus (1493–1541), and Nicholas Culpeper (1616–1654). Humoral medicine is currently experiencing a resurgence in British folk medicine, as revived by Christopher Hedley, evolved and tweaked for modern times.

I want to know about the visible fluids and don't hesitate to ask my clients about their bowel movements, their color and mucous content, and general gassiness. I'll also ask about the length of their bleeding times, in cuts and injuries, as well as menstrual bleeding, or the color of their urine. Understanding the movement of the major body fluids and what constitutes healthy fluids can be important in assessing health patterns.

The influence of humoral medicine on the folk medicine of the South cannot be overstated.

As we discuss the concepts of Southern Folk Medicine, it seems evident that the humoral system of Europe, in its form at the time of settlement of the New World, met and intertwined with the Indigenous folk medicines and uses of medicinal plants of the New World (which could also technically be called humoral systems). This melding occurred not only in the Southeastern United States, but also in Mexico, the Caribbean, and South America—other areas which the Spanish explored and conquered.

A Quick Overview of the Humoral System

The humoral system's primary concept is that both health and disease are influenced by the complex interactions among a person's four humors. These interactions are affected by their lifestyle, diet, habits, emotional stability, and environment. Therapeutic approaches based on an individualized assessment can help bring balance to the humoral makeup.

Any humoral system, whether Greek, Native American, Southern Folk Medicine, Traditional Chinese Medicine, or Ayurveda, which developed in a time when people lived close to the Earth and used a language based on local climate, topography, and land, will have some similarities. Folks depended upon the land for their food, clothing, and shelter. The lives of the people were totally entwined with every aspect of living on the land, and for this reason, they used a land-based vocabulary. The vocabulary forms the basis of most all folk medicines regardless of cultural origin.

The four humors are blood, phlegm, bile, and black bile. While three of the four relate quite easily to body fluids, the fourth, black bile, has been defined alternately as toxins, necrosis, or excrement—basically, all the nasty stuff. All humors were believed to be made by the liver from digestion of food—which isn't a far stretch when you think about the role the liver plays in the digestive process, methylation, and metabolism of all substances we take into our bodies.

The four humors form in the body and move through it. With the humors in balance, a person is healthy; an imbalance of any of the humors causes illness. To return to health, a balance of humors must be reinstated. This is a continual process since the humors are in perpetual motion. Humors are affected by a person's mental and physical health, and also their disposition.

In the humoral model, an excess or deficiency of one or more humors results in imbalance and illness. The excess or deficiency is assessed within a person's individual constitution. Almost anything could shift a humor to excess or deficiency: too much wine, not enough food, too little exercise, too much exercise, not enough sleep, working in a toxic environment, a fight with your lover, or the death of a loved one. According to Hippocrates, the humors could be brought back into balance by targeted nutrition and lifestyle changes. Galen added the use of medicinal herbs as a therapeutic approach and categorized the herbs into a useful system for ease of use.

The four humors or fluids corresponded to the four elements of Greek philosophy—fire, water, air, and earth—these four elements composed all matter, each with a specific characteristic. Earth is solid and heavy and flows downward, collecting in the feet, legs, bowels, and abdomen. Water is liquid and heavy and flows downward, collecting in the same areas as earth. Wind or air is gassy and light, and flows upward and outward, though it may move around the lower body without pattern. Fire flows upward and out, but burns in the digestive tract and reproductive organs.

Within the humoral system—based on the Greeks' Mediterranean environment—yellow bile is considered hot and dry, like fire upon the land. Phlegm is considered cold and wet, like swampy water. Blood is considered hot and wet, like the air coming in from the Mediterranean Sea. And black bile is considered cold and dry, like the dirt beneath the surface of the land or within a Mediterranean cave. Because health and the humors are connected to the land, certain seasons of the year then influence the movement of the humors around the body.

Hot, cold, and warm are humoral values used to describe an analogical quality that can be applied to food, herbs, remedies, physical conditions, and temperaments, as well as thermal temperatures. This is also true of the humoral qualities of wet, dry, moist, hard, soft, rising, falling, high, low, thick, and thin, and other qualities used also in Southern Folk Medicine.

The qualities—hot, cold, wet, dry—result from opposing characteristics of the humors. This paring of opposite qualities is very influential in Southern Folk Medicine: hot/cold; wet/dry. For example, phlegm is cold and moist while blood is hot and moist. The qualities of the humor then influence the temperaments: sanguine (blood), choleric (bile), phlegmatic (phlegm), or melancholic (black bile). Temperaments not only describe physical complaints or symptoms but also personality and emotional outlook. They are assessed by several physical and psychological markers, including physical characteristics of the face and skin, as well as personality traits.

The temperaments are ever-changing and interact with each other. For example, if a substance becomes too hot, it can also become dry. These four basic temperaments can combine in various ways to create sixteen different combinations of temperaments that can be measured by observation and assessment.

The humors influence the temperaments. Blood is hot and moist; phlegm is cold and moist; bile is hot and dry; and black bile is cold and dry. When the humors are in balance, Vital Energy is strong and the body is healthy. In humoral medicine, each body fluid is associated with an emotion: blood (sanguine, happy, creative); phlegm (satisfied, dull, lazy); bile (choleric, ambitious, energetic); and black bile (melancholic, introverted, self-pitying).

The equivalent of a temperament in Southern Folk Medicine is the constitution. Understanding the personality and physical makeup of a constitution is an important assessment tool for herbalists and healers in Southern Folk Medicine. Rather than the imbalance being considered the cause, it's the observation of the fluids that is important for seeing markers or signs of an imbalance that needs addressing.

For a deeper understanding of humoral medicine in modern days, I refer you to *The Traditional Healer's Handbook* (1991) by Hakim G.M. Chishti. Matthew Wood, a well-known herbalist from Minnesota, has written extensively on the humoral system in several of his books and a number of articles. Christopher Hedley, an herbalist in London, has done much to revitalize humoral medicine in modern-day herbalism in Britain.

The four humors, and the humoral language, were such a normal part of Elizabethan English life that their influence can be seen in Shakespeare's plays and sonnets. He uses the language of the four humors to describe the personalities of his characters, their physical form, and their psychological motivations. What may be even more remarkable is that Shakespeare's audience understood his words perfectly through the lens of the four humors—the humoral language was that common! I would also like to note that Elizabeth I was queen of England at the time of the first discoveries of the New World, and her successor, James I, authorized the translation of the King James Bible that so influenced Southern Folk Medicine and Christianity in the New World. That version of the Bible is also filled with humoral language.

Once we earnestly begin our introduction into Southern Folk Medicine, the influence of the basic principles of the humoral system will be quite obvious. Yet there will be pronounced differences as well.

I leave this discussion with a quote from Shakespeare's *Hamlet* (melancholy, black bile): "I have of late, but wherefore I know not, lost all my mirth, forgone all custom of exercises; and indeed, it goes so heavily with my disposition that this goodly frame, the earth, seems to me a most sterile promontory; this most excellent canopy, the air, look you, this brave o'er hanging firmament, this majestical roof fretted golden fire: why it appeareth nothing to me but a foul and pestilent congregation of vapors…. Man delights me not; nor woman neither."

Native American Influence

While the humoral medicine of the Old World is a major influence on Southern Folk Medicine, it is just one. Without the ability to utilize the native plants of the New World, settlers would have been missing the most important tool of the healing arts—the herbs themselves. Although some food and medicinal plants from Europe arrived with the colonists, they soon had to turn to local plants to survive. Local plants were also economically important as new medicines and ornamentals that could be a source of trade in the home country.

Plants that made the journey from Europe and became naturalized—dandelion, cleavers, chickweed, calendula, elecampane, red clover, alfalfa, and mullein to name a few—soon spread from the gardens of the settlers into the local environment, and are now common in herbalists' materia medica. Red clover can now be found growing wild in all of North America. It's everywhere! These naturalized plants have become so common that many modern herbalists don't fully understand their unique properties and use them more as beverage teas.

The know-how to use local, native plants was gleaned from Indigenous peoples by settlers, indentured servants, and slaves. Here in the South, the Creeks (Muskogee) and the Cherokees (Tsalagi) were the primary tribes that interacted with the white invaders. Native Americans were often reluctant to share health practices with the white man simply because many health practices were also considered spiritual practices. Native remedies that were shared with the white man were the more commonly used herbal ones that many people in the tribe might know. Spiritual practices, on the other hand, were sacred knowledge that only a few might possess. A vast number of the native Eastern woodland plants used in modern herbalism are based on this greater shared knowledge. We owe a huge debt to Native Americans for our current ability to use native plants effectively.

As in humoral medicine, the cosmology of Native Americans in the Southeast includes four elements—fire, water, wind or air, and earth. The elements were linked to each of the four cardinal directions—north, south, east, and west. It is truly amazing how often these same basic four elements are a part of the healing practices of so many different cultures around the world, especially considering that these cultures didn't interact with each other, held very different religious beliefs, and were continents apart.

In Creek medicine, for greatest effect, every herbal formula contained all four elements. Also in Creek society, special healers and protectors of the tribe mastered the elements and could call upon them at will. Mastering wind was considered an especially useful talent to manage the tornadoes that often ravaged the area. It was also useful to be able to send a storm against an enemy during a battle or use wind for protection.

Each element had a specific purpose in Native health practice. Water is rejuvenating and cleansing, and represents purity. This is one of the reasons prayers are often performed at water. The wind carries sound, not only between peoples but also between Great Mystery and people. Fire is so important to Native Peoples that after much training, some people are designated Fire Keepers. It represents transformation and the feminine, as well as the sun on Earth. Fire is symbolized by the thunderbolt; lightning strikes the land and fire results. And finally, the Earth is the mother of us all; all things growing or dug from the Earth are considered earthen and a gift from our common mother.

A fifth element sometimes appears in Southeast Native American cosmology. It might be called Great Mystery, Great Spirit, or Emptiness. It has been described as the invisible spirit that connects the Earth to the sky, or that which binds all things together.

Native views of sickness and health also took into account the importance of relationship—to Spirit, to tribe, to family, and to self. Imbalances in any relationship or any prolonged conflict in relationships could cause illness. While specific healing techniques were based on the regional practices of the tribes, some generalities can be found among the healing practices and philosophies of the tribes of the Southeast. David Winston has summarized seven core areas of knowledge required by Native healers.

According to Winston (2001), "a core of indigenous belief [Cherokee}]and plant use remains today." He further states that the Native healer must master seven interconnected areas of knowledge: herb use (medicinal and ceremonial) and personality of the plants; physical medicine, including midwifery, minor surgery, moxibustion, and persimmon wood stampers; dream interpretation, for personal growth, healing, and to gain knowledge; language/myths/laws; ceremonies; laws of nature; and conjuring (magic, spells).While Winston speaks particularly of the Cherokee, these seven areas of healing knowledge can be generalized for any of the Five Civilized Tribes of the Southeast: the Creek, Cherokee, Choctaw, Chickasaw, and Seminole tribes.

Native Americans who had not been forcibly removed from the South during the ethnic cleansing known as the Trail of Tears (1831–1839) continued to have a strong influence on Southern Folk Medicine. Some traditional Native medicine ways were remembered, but many more were lost or diluted by time and with continued contact with the dominant white culture. Native Americans who remained behind were often the healers and herbalists for the poor white and black communities.

Though many medicine ways had been lost, the use of native medicinal plants continued to be taught within the remaining pockets of Native culture for many generations. My own grandmother, Rosie Light, who claimed Creek descent, was one such person. In her youth, she helped deliver babies and gather and dispense herbs to a community of poor that had no money for doctors.

Native healers were considered excellent herbalists and their services were sought after. The herbs they used were considered to be of higher quality than the average store-bought herb. This belief in the quality of Native American herbs and practices continues to this day, so much so that the word "Indian" on a bottle of herbs or on products sold as "Indian remedies" definitely helps increase sales in the South and elsewhere.

According to James Mooney in *The Swimmer Manuscript: Cherokee Sacred Formulas and Medicinal Prescriptions,* there were two broad causes of disease: natural or supernatural. Mooney writes, "However primitive and unsophisticated may be the views of a tribe on disease and its causes, and however great may be the share of mysticism and occultism in its explanation of the events of daily life, yet there is almost everywhere a recognition of natural agency if not for some of the ailments, at least for some accidents."

Mooney writes of supernatural causes of disease, "If even in cases where the natural course and cause of events seems evident and obvious, a mythologic explanation may be advanced, what are we to expect when it becomes necessary to account for such mysterious, unexplainable, insidious changes of condition to which disease subjects our body and mind?"

The causes of illness—natural, supernatural, and magical—of the Southeastern natives found their way into Southern Folk Medicine and Hoodoo. From the perspective of Southern Folk Medicine, this will be discussed in greater detail in a following chapter. But I do want to acknowledge at this time that these categories were used by the natives prior to contact with whites.

Spirits may also cause disease. The Cherokee believed in a multitude of spirits, mostly animal spirits, which could also cause disease. Mooney writes, "As a rule the spirit who has caused a disease is never prevailed upon to take the disease away; the office of another, rival, spirit is called upon to do this. Spirits do not merely send disease of their own initiative; they may be prevailed upon to do so by human agency, by witches or by man killers, for instance."

The most important, the most powerful spirit was Great Mystery, which missionaries dubbed the Great Spirit or Creator. This spirit was often identified with the sun and was considered feminine, while another spirit, which was identified with the moon, was considered masculine. The sun was often referred to as "grandmother." Rarely did the sun cause disease, but rather she was often called upon by prayer to cure disease. The sun was associated with fire: "the medicine man warms his hands over these coals before he starts 'rubbing the disease away.'" Fire was also used to create decoctions that were either taken internally or rubbed on the body.

According to Mooney, the moon, often referred to as "grandfather," was not associated with any illness, but acknowledging the moon in all its cycles was a way to ward off illness. The river, water, could also send disease to those who disrespected it by throwing in rubbish or urinating in it. Many rituals of the Cherokees were also performed at water, usually at daybreak. Ghosts can also cause illness, especially those of slain animals or humans. Ghosts may reincarnate in another body, whether animal or human, each in their original form, until such a time that their cycle is finished.

Magical causes of illness include those affected by witches, which can be male or female. Mooney writes, "Moreover, whatever the witch can steal of the life, and therefore of the vital principle, of the animus, the power, the 'orenda' of its victim, he adds to his own, and this is the reason why witches are always hovering about the sick, the feeble, the moribund people; invisible as they can make themselves, they put their mouths over those of the victims, and steal their breath; according to some informants 'because they like the taste of sick people's breath; it is so sweet'; according to others, because stealing their breath comes to the same as securing for themselves the victim's vitality, which they add to their own. At the time the moribund expires, especially, the witch is careful not to miss his chance." A sick person often had family members or friends watching during the night to protect from witchcraft. Burning tobacco could keep away the witch.

In the Cherokee tradition, there are other influences of health and illness, too many for the scope of this book, including dreams and neglecting taboos. It was the intent of the healer to remove the cause of the illness, not manage the illness, and to this end, much investigation and questioning occurred, including using dreams as an assessment tool and questioning about family life. This approach definitely made its way into Southern Folk Medicine, as we'll discuss later.

Native Americans had no remedies for the illnesses brought by the settlers. Measles, mumps, chicken pox, small pox, venereal disease, and tuberculosis took the lives of thousands and thousands of Native Americans who had never been exposed to those viruses or bacteria and therefore did not have any innate immunity against the pathogens. They reasoned that white man's medicine was needed to treat white man's diseases. To this end, Native healers were quick to learn the new invasive plants and how to use them. For example, according to the

Encyclopedia of Cultivated Plants: From Acacia to Zinnia, edited by Christopher Cumo, "mullein quickly gained a foothold with Native American cultures who adopted it for a number of uses," including tuberculosis. Other plants included catnip, chickweed, plantain, peppermint, Queen Anne's lace, yarrow, elecampane, red clover, alfalfa, and dandelion.

The more well-known native plants and their medicinal or food uses that were used by Native populations are too numerous to list in this short space, but I must mention a few that have continued to be used by herbalists today: black cohosh, blue cohosh, partridge berry, bay laurel, magnolia, dogwood, sycamore, tulip poplar, blue vervain, boneset, sassafras, sarsaparilla, black walnut, cayenne, corn silk, evening primrose, birch, goldenseal, American ginseng, fringetree, elderberry, echinacea, hydrangea, juniper berry, cedar berry, lobelia, poke, gravel root, prickly ash, red root, raspberry, pinkroot, skullcap, Solomon's seal, spicebush, white pine, wild indigo, mayapple, bloodroot, angelica, osha, angelica, wild cherry, wild yam, yellow root, pipsissewa, huckleberry, rabbit tobacco, tag alder, sumac, sweetgum, and smartweed. Whew! A nice little list.

The Trail of Tears

The Trail of Tears played an important role in the ancestral lineage and herbal legacy of many folks in north Alabama and across the Southeast, including me. Though much has been written about the forcible removal of the Cherokees from North Carolina, I must add that all Southeast natives were removed including the Choctaws, Alabamas, Creeks, Hitachi, Seminole, Yuchi, and Chickasaw. Whites wanted the land in the Southern states to grow cotton, for it was in planting cotton that fortunes were made. Also, in 1828, gold was discovered near present-day Dahlonega, Georgia, on Cherokee land. This small gold rush was the added impetus to remove the remaining Cherokee. President Andrew Jackson drafted the Indian Removal Act in 1830, which paved the way for the Trail of Tears.

In 1831, the Choctaw became the first nation to be expelled from their land and made the journey to Indian territory on foot, often bound in chains and without any food, supplies, or other help from the government. Thousands of people died along the way. It was, one Choctaw leader told an Alabama newspaper, a "trail of tears and death." Thus was named the forced march. The rounding up and removing of Native peoples continued slowly until 1836 to 1838, when the process was sped up by the U.S. government.

In 1836, leaving from Gunter's Landing, Alabama, several thousand Creeks were forced to their new home. Many of these Creeks had been living with the Cherokees and were rounded up from Alabama to North Carolina. In 1838, the first group of Cherokees also made the long trip. They attempted to take the water route down the Tennessee River, which was in drought so that the barges couldn't float.

The natives were sent to base camps at various points around the Southeast. From the base camps, the natives were sent to detention camps at emigration points along the Singing (Tennessee) River. One such detention camp was at Gunter's Landing at the big bend of the river at present day Guntersville, Alabama. The Tennessee River flows across the entire state of Alabama, entering in the northeast corner of the state and exiting at the western corner near Waterloo.

During the drought, several hundred natives escaped into the hills and hollows of north Alabama where these "deserters" found a new home in a relatively sparsely populated land. For this reason, North Alabama has a rich Native American heritage. According to the website of the Echota Cherokee Tribe of Alabama, "The members of the Echota Cherokee Tribe of Alabama are the descendants of those Indian people who escaped the infamous 'Trail of Tears' by hiding out in the mountainous backwoods and lowlands of the Southeast. Others fled from the march after it began and others simply walked away and came home after reaching Indian Territory. They kept to themselves, did not speak the language, and did not teach it to their children for fear the child might speak it in the presence of someone who would learn the secret of their ancestry. If this happened, they could immediately be taken into custody and sent to Indian Territory in the west. Everything they owned could be given away by the state."

The fear of being sent to Indian Territory in the West was a very tangible one that I remember from my childhood. This very situation happened to a family member and became one of the stories within the Light family. And it was this fear that encouraged natives to take care of their own during sickness with the use of local herbs and traditional healing techniques. Though many of the healing stories were lost, the use of local herbs remained, and this information was often shared within local communities, thus adding to the richness of Southern Folk Medicine.

African-American Influence

Slavery did not begin in the New World, but its institution affected the development of countries and cultures in a way that was unprecedented in history. The first slaves to the New World were Moors brought by the Spanish, first to the coast of what later became South Carolina in 1526, by Lucas Vasquez de Ayllon, and also to Florida in 1565, by Admiral Don Pedro Menendez de Aviles. Moorish slaves, generally from North Africa, had been used by the Spanish and much of the Middle East and Mediterranean countries for several hundred years. Moorish slaves were highly skilled craftsman and artisans who were brought to help build houses, forts, and defensive walls, as well as to take care of their masters. During Spain's history, slaves could be African, Moorish, or Christian, depending upon who was in power. When Muslims were in power, Christians were slaves, and when Christians were in power, then Moors were slaves. At the time of settlement of the New World, Christians were in power in Spain.

Spain initially tried to use Native Americans as slaves, but this wasn't successful. Natives were not familiar with the building techniques which the Spanish required, ran away whenever possible, and died in droves from European diseases. There was also the religious issue of using Native Americans as slaves (but not Africans or whites), and ultimately in 1542, Charles V, Holy Roman Emperor, decreed that natives could not be used as slaves. It would be many years before this decree reached full fruition in regard to Native peoples.

The Spanish slave trade began in earnest when Portuguese slave traders brought several hundred African slaves to Spain. The Portuguese had been trading slaves to the West Indies, Hispaniola, and South America since about 1510, and had been actively trading in Europe since about 1450. By the sixteenth century, the majority of slaves in Spain, as well as those going to the Spanish Caribbean and Cuba to work in the sugar cane fields, were of African descent.

The Dutch, who also supplied African slaves to the Spanish New World, initiated the North American slave trade when they brought eleven African slaves from the West Indies to what is now New York in 1626.

The peoples of northern and western Africa who came willingly or unwillingly to the American South contributed an amazing spiritual framework to the folk medicine that survives today. Africa also contributed several foods that are now considered a staple of Southern cooking. The most common of these are okra, rice, black-eyed peas, sorghum, watermelons, and yams. These foods were brought aboard the ships to feed the Africans on the long voyage. Food that was leftover and seeds that were saved were planted by the slaves upon arrival in the South. Foods common in Southern cooking such as pinto, kidney, red, navy, black, and Great Northern beans, sweet potatoes, peanuts, and hominy are actually New World foods.

Initially, African slaves to the New World (North and South America) were males who had been slaves in Africa. Later males who were captured in war, were local criminals, or had been captured to sell were sent to the Americas. Slaves brought from West and Central Africa worked in agriculture, in the cultivation of tobacco and cotton, and in the milling of sugar and as domestic labor. Later, African women were brought as slaves and to become breeding stock for future generations of bound peoples. Children that were brought were generally sent to the Caribbean.

By 1850, most of the slaves in the United States were third-, fourth-, or fifth generation Americans, and far removed from Africa. Ninety percent of Africans brought to the New World as slaves went to the Caribbean and South America, not North America.

I've searched and searched for documentation of medicinal plants brought from Africa with the slaves, and there just doesn't seem to be any. There is documentation that some Africans braided licorice seeds in their hair, but one conjecture was that the licorice seeds made the hair smell sweet and was attractive to the opposite sex. As far as my research has uncovered, the Africans who were taken or sold as slaves could not bring their medicine, their plants, or their healers with them. What they could bring were their healing framework of how to use herbs, rituals, customs, and their music and dances.

And, what could these people do once they were here? How could they survive? They could do what anyone in such a horrible situation would—the best they could with what they had. This included learning information from Native Americans about local plants, and learning information about herbs from other indentured servants and slaves who were carrying forth the information in oral form. It also meant taking aspects of other cultural groups (Native American, Scottish, Irish, Spanish, French, German, and English) and making something unique.

In those days, people passed on the practice of folk medicine as an oral tradition, often dropping out tidbits and gems of information in normal conversation.

There were some common health remedies that everyone was expected to know as part of the normal cultural experience. A person had to know and be able to use a certain amount of health and herbal information in order to survive. Times were hard and lean, and everyone depended upon the land and its resources for life and livelihood. This commonality helped create movement of healthcare information across economic and social lines.

As Sharla M. Fett writes in *Working Cures,* fluidity of healthcare information had been in practice since the beginning of the country. Even in the antebellum South, people sought "effective medicines and skilled practitioners across lines of social division. Therapies circulated with surprising fluidity as health seekers turned to Thomsonianism, homeopathy, water cure, Indian remedies, and Hoodoo." The willingness to move across social lines for healthcare information is still the norm today. Southerners from all economic stations of life are quite comfortable consulting herbalists, seers, scripture, energy healers, almanacs, and the information passed around in family, church groups, and neighborhoods.

From the very beginning of their experiences in North America, African slaves faced daunting health issues. Often their masters seemed to be virtually indifferent as to whether they survived or perished. Logically to modern sensibilities, it would seem that slave owners, for economic and humanitarian reasons, would have maintained their human property in healthy, working order, but that wasn't always the case, especially in the Caribbean. The horrendous conditions on slave ships, where astoundingly large numbers of Africans died before ever reaching North America, showed that slave traders often didn't value the slaves despite their monetary value.

According to Iain Gately, author of *Tobacco,* the "received wisdom" at many sugar plantations in the early British colonies was that it was beneficial to simply work slaves to death. Consequently, as he points out, the number of slaves in Barbados barely increased by 25,000 during the first fifty years of the eighteenth century, despite the fact that during that time over 150,000 slaves had been shipped to the island. Later, on the mainland of North America, conditions for slaves marginally improved as owners saw the economic advantages of letting them survive long enough to have children. As Gately notes, for many farmers, the value of their slaves represented their largest single investment; in contrast, the land they cultivated was relatively inexpensive.

During the antebellum South, an early conceptual conflict arose around the different definitions of health between the owner and the slaves. The idea of health and happiness for slaves was severely limited by their servitude and life experiences. Slaves were also restricted, bound in their healing experiences and practices, by how much latitude their owners permitted in the use of herbs and other healing techniques. Some owners permitted slaves to choose their own remedies, which fostered a sense of independence for the slaves and the appearance of some control over their lives. Other owners refused to allow their slaves to learn about herbs, fearing that the knowledge of plants and poisons might be turned against them. And some owners called in white doctors to treat their slaves.

Medical knowledge, science, herb use, religion, and conjuring often clashed on the plantation because of different views held by slaves and owners over both the causes of illness and treatment of the sick. African-American slaves believed that physical illness could be caused by curses, conjuring, or spiritual degradation, and often viewed medical help offered by white doctors as worthless. White conventional doctors did not believe that illness could be caused by emotions or spirits.

In addition to the influence on Southern Folk Medicine, the coming together of Celtic culture and Africa in the South produced other amazing contributions to American culture: in music, the creation or influence on jazz, bluegrass, rhythm and blues, rock and roll, hip-hop, country music, ragtime, boogie woogie, rap, soul, and pop songs; in dance, the creation or influence on tap, jazz dance, buck dance, stick dances, swing, jitterbug, juke joint dancing, break dance, and hip-hop. Oh, and let's not forget the banjo. What would bluegrass be without the banjo?

The Irish and British Isles

The Irish arrived much earlier in the New World than is taught in most public schools. According to Donald Harman Akenson, author of *If the Irish Ran the World: Montserrat, 1630–1730,* "The first significant number of Irishmen to serve the European powers in the Western Hemisphere seem to have been part of the Spanish garrison in Florida in the mid-1560s." Irish priests also came with Spanish explorers, and an Irish priest served the city of St. Augustine from 1598 to 1606. The Irish count, Arthur O'Neil, was the Spanish governor of West Florida beginning in 1781. Historical sources also believe that Irish soldiers served with Spanish explorers in the late 1500s. Whether these soldiers interacted with local natives is unknown.

Britain was late to settle the New World. By the time the British sought to stake a claim here, the Swedish and Dutch had already joined the Spanish and French in claiming land. Britain was slow to move due to internal religious strife and turmoil, and the extreme poverty of the nation. In addition, early attempts at colonization had proved disastrous, including the lost colony of Roanoke in 1585, and sparked little interest in the potential for further monetary loss.

British colonies, unlike the Spanish and French, which were funded almost exclusively by the monarchies, were funded in a variety of ways. There were the joint-stock companies, which sold stock in the colonies to investors; these charter companies were a forerunner of the modern corporation. There were crown or royal colonies, which were under the direct rule of a governor appointed by the monarchy. And there were also proprietary colonies given as rewards to friends and allies of the British monarchy.

Expeditions to the New World were often led by minor sons of well-to-do families, wealthy merchants, and, in the northeast, by the Puritans. British venturers searched futilely for gold and precious gems. It was, for the British, an herb that finally created the wealth they sought. Growing tobacco, which required a large labor force, was the first profitable investment by the British in the New World. Indentured servants, both British and Irish, were brought to grow tobacco in the South and the British Caribbean Islands.

Initially, indentured servants brought by the British were generally young, single, indentured Irish men, and British landless and convicts. There was a great need for strong labor to clear and tend vast amounts of acreage. Indentured servants worked a limited number of years, usually seven, and were then given their freedom. Although indentured servitude was harsh, it was not slavery, and many people willingly indentured themselves for the opportunity for a more prosperous life in the New World. Ultimately, the number of indentured servants, who came willingly or unwillingly to the New World, could not keep up with the demand for labor. In addition, freed indentured servants often became competition for their previous masters. For these reasons, by the late 1600s, black slaves were beginning to fill the gaps in the labor force.

Britain used the New World as a penal colony for convicts and criminals to work off their sentences. It's estimated that at least half-a-million indentured servants went to British holdings in the Caribbean. The New World was also a pressure valve to relieve the overpopulated British Isles, which boasted a huge poor and landless population. Whole families immigrated to the Northeast seeking a better life. Britain was also at war with Spain, and settling the New World was seen as a way to extend their rivalry on other shores.

By 1620, the Virginia Company of London was exporting only one crop—tobacco. According to Thomas Hariot in *A Briefe and True Report of the New Found Land of Virginia* (1588): "Its leaves are dried, made into powder, and then smoked by being sucked through clay pipes into the stomach and head. The fumes purge superfluous phlegm and gross humors from the body by opening all the pores and passages. Thus its use not only preserves the body, but if there are any obstructions it breaks them up. By this means the natives are kept in excellent health, without many of the grievous diseases which often afflict us in England." By 1630, over one million pounds of tobacco were being exported from Virginia annually.

The New World also helped provide a solution for the British to the Irish problem. The Irish were removed from the British Isles in even greater number than British landless and convicts. Beginning in 1490, and continuing in four waves through 1603, England undertook an ethnic cleansing of the Irish, especially of Irish Catholics, in order to vacate lands for Protestant landowners and English and Scottish tenant farmers. The Irish were forced off the land, often emigrating to France or Spain and the British Caribbean islands. Ultimately, English landowners had trouble finding English or Scottish tenants to work the land and eventually returned to using Irish tenants. This was known as the Plantation period, and it was this Plantation model that the English later brought to the Southern United States to grow cotton and tobacco.

Initially, hundreds of Irish either voluntarily left Ireland or were banished. Whole clans left to avoid death or servitude. Irish families followed their chieftains into exile, bringing with them their healers, to settle in the New World or Europe. It is this fact, that the Irish who left voluntarily brought their healers, that is unique in its influence on Southern and Caribbean Folk Medicine. The exodus of healers and seers from Ireland left the remaining Irish people with reduced medical care and a reduced traditional Irish folk medicine.

The practice of Irish indentured servitude in the British New World continued through the reigns of James I and II and through Charles I, but it was Oliver Cromwell who devastated the Irish population. Farm workers, Irish beggars, criminals, and orphans were also indentured to the New World. Although the exact numbers of Irish men, women, and children who were indentured to North America and the Caribbean as forced labor is greatly debated, there is no doubt that this grievous situation existed. Through either death, forced removal, or famine, the population of Ireland fell from 1,500,000 to about 600,000.

The majority of the Irish who came to the British New World as indentured servants or felons went to the Caribbean. According to Grady McWhiney, in *Cracker Culture,* "By the time of the Restoration, Irish constituted a large majority of the perhaps 80,000 white inhabitants of the English islands in the Caribbean. Barbados had, at that time, about 30,000 black slaves and about 20,000 indentured white felons and rebels, these being overwhelmingly Irish; St. Christopher was said to contain 20,000 Irish." Today, about 30 percent of the population of Montserrat have Irish surnames. Beginning in 1669, the Irish labor force in the Caribbean was being replaced by black slaves from Africa.

As Irish indentured servants in the Caribbean were freed, many made their way into the Gulf of Mexico or along the southern Atlantic coast, and from there contributed to the large number of Irish in the South, exploring and settling from the southern shore upward.

According to McWhiney, by 1640, more than 5,000 Irish had settled in Virginia, either by emigration, as indentured servants, felons, or rebels, or had been kidnapped and sent to the New World. Between 1720 and 1760, around 30,000 Irish arrived in Maryland and Virginia as convicts. By 1790, it is estimated that the Irish comprised 25 percent of the population of South Carolina and 27 percent of the population of Georgia. As Irish servants worked off their freedom in Virginia, they moved further south into the Carolinas, Tennessee, Alabama, and Georgia. This trend continued through the migration of the Scotch-Irish in the 1750s and happened again in the 1840s.

The Scotch-Irish didn't arrive in the South until the late 1700s, and the largest wave arrived in the decades prior to the Civil War, around 1839. Along with their energy and independence, they also brought their own view of health and a unique system of healthcare based on hundreds of years of living in a cold, damp land.

Later waves of free Scotch-Irish came in droves to ports in the northeast and filtered down into the Appalachian mountains, seeking the independence promised in a new land.

During this later Irish emigration, whole families left Ireland in hopes of acquiring land, a situation that was patently impossible back home. They brought much of their folk medicine and cultural constructs with them, in a much more traceable manner than Africans were able to do.

Being of a clannish nature, early Celts to the South intermarried regularly with Native Americans. Marriages with natives helped facilitate the acceptance of white settlers in the area, gave them authority in local European government, and helped them receive large land grants. Many important Southern families began their land empires by marrying into local tribes—Creeks, Cherokees, Choctaws, and Chickasaws. These intermarriages produced such prominent Native chiefs as William Mcintosh and Alexander McGillivray of the Creek and William Hicks and John Looney of the Cherokee.

Other ways in which Irish folk medicine influenced Southern Folk Medicine are both practical and superstitious. Lard, or pig grease, was the most common medium for salve making in Ireland and became so in the South. In the early days, almost every community in the South had a bonesetter, and so did the communities in Ireland. In Ireland, the position of healer or herbalist was generally an inherited one, and information and knowledge stayed within families. The same is true in parts of the South. Both Tommie Bass's parents were knowledgeable herbalists, and their salve recipe had been brought by the family from the British Isles. My initial teachings came from my grandmother and father, who carried down information through the generations.

Irish folk medicine practices often contained a ritual with a Christian element. In Southern Folk Medicine, this is also true. Talking off warts, blowing fire, or stopping blood usually consists of an action, an herb, and a prayer or Bible verse. And let's not forget prayer and faith healing. The bowl of Irish oat mush and milk became, in the South, crumbled cornbread and milk or grits and milk. Scotch whiskey from barley became bourbon made from corn.

The Irish and Scotch-Irish had already integrated Christianity into their healing system when they arrived in the New World—Christianity and superstition often went hand in hand for these immigrants. The duality of Irish and Scotch-Irish folk practices can be seen in the use of moon signs, astrology, and the view that spiritual actions could cause illness, a view also held by Africans. These concepts greatly impacted Southern Folk Medicine.

The Irish folk system, much like the Native American one, also viewed illnesses as either "natural" or "unnatural." Here is a passage from the *Rosa Anglica*, which was probably written in 1314. I quote the English translation from the fourth printed edition, Augsburg, 1595, discussing both natural and unnatural fevers: "Fever is the same as natural heat turning to fieriness, according to Hippocrates and Galen....This is tertian fever, unnatural heat generated from increase of choler which afflicts every action...." As you can see, the humoral or Greek system of medicine was quite entrenched in Ireland before the 1300s.

From the *Rosa Anglica*, a sure cure for warts: "Item take burnt willow bark and mix it with vinegar; this will cure warts on being applied to them." I would like to point out that willow bark contains salicylic acid, the same compound that is found in many over-the-counter wart remedies today. Also, vinegar is still an excellent home remedy for removing warts. In the *Rosa Anglica*, both remedies are combined, which should give excellent results. The text also mentions using cobwebs or spider webs to stop the flow of blood, which is another traditional Appalachian remedy.

Economic ways also emigrated from Ireland to the South. By the Civil War, more than half the men in the South did not own any land, which was concentrated in the hands of the few, much like in Ireland during the times of immigration. This is a pattern that continued in the South. Fischer writes in *Albion's Seed*, "In 1983, the top 1 percent of owners possessed half of the land in Appalachia. The top 5 percent owned nearly two-thirds. This pattern of wealth distribution...in the twentieth century was much like that which had existed two hundred years earlier."

Regional Isolation, War, and Depression

The massive plantation culture brought to the New World by the English served to isolate and separate the peoples of the South from the rest of the country in very significant ways. The isolation of the poor whites, slaves, and Native Americans from conventional society nurtured the Southern Folk Medicine and allowed it to evolve unhindered from outside influences for generations.

By the first part of the nineteenth century, slavery in the South was largely confined to rural areas where every inch of fertile, flat land was planted with cotton. The isolation of the plantations made supervision of the slaves easy. National laws against the slave trade slowed the flow of Africans into the South but did not abolish slavery. After 1810, most slaves were born in North America, a truly American culture, often the descendants of families that had been in this country longer than their owners.

A look at the class makeup in the pre–Civil War era and immediately follow-ing the war allows a glimpse of understanding into the continued development of Southern Folk Medicine. During this time, the South was divided into various classes of white Christians; at one extreme were the landowners (planters) and at the other extreme were the poor whites (non–land owners, non-merchants), who, in the lowly vernacular, were called "white trash" or "crackers." Unless they were indentured servants, poor whites were excluded from working on planta-tions alongside the slaves because of the color of their skin. Poor whites were uneducated, and this prevented them from any economic opportunity. The people in these poor white communities were as isolated from society as those on the plantations, but in a different way. Those closest to the poor whites in social status were the slaves. These two groups interacted and shared informa-tion, but were also antagonistic toward each other, a situation encouraged by the wealthy. The isolation of the poor whites from the rest of white society helped nurture local folk medicine, a healing system not bound to the communities of poor whites or blacks, but one which flourished in each and traveled across racial and economic lines.

The path which folk medicine evolved from—interactions among slaves, their owners, and Native Americans—shows that a wide variety of influences were at work. For example, in *Working Cures*, Fett discusses an 1855 letter writ-ten by William Berly, a planter from South Carolina, who was looking for ways to treat his father's intestinal ailments. In the letter, Mr. Berly explains how to use a weed called opossum ear. Boiled in port wine, this plant made a medi-cine that offered digestive relief. Mr. Berly reveals that he obtained information about opossum ear from a Mr. Wingard, one of his white neighbors. This Native American treatment had been communicated to Mr. Wingard by "his old negro Sam." Sam, in turn, had been taught about the herb by a man from New Orleans who had got his knowledge from an "Indian doctor." As Ms. Fett, notes, this type of complex web of knowledge of folk medicine demonstrates a "complex history where remedies were borrowed, purchased, and stolen to create overlapping traditions of southern herbalism."

The Civil War saw the spread of folk herbalism out of the domain of the poor whites, Native Americans, and slaves into the middle and upper classes. The South was in a blockade and few medicines were able to cross the blockade lines except through the black market. During this time, Southern Folk Medicine found acceptance among physicians and pharmacists, who began to codify the use of the native plants into a more conventional medicine language. There were scant medical supplies available to the Confederate Army physicians, which often sent them searching in the fields and forests for herbal aids.

Some writers of Civil War history consider the physician's folk use of herbs for battlefield injuries and seasoning diseases to be innovative and creative. It was really desperation. There were literally few conventional medicines available and folk medicines were easy to find. The Civil War served to bring elements of Southern Folk Medicine into the mainstream, where it has stayed, to some extent, ever since.

One of the most important books from that time period was *Resources of the Southern Fields and Forests, Medical, Economical, and Agricultural: Being Also a Medical Botany of the Confederate States; with Practical Information on the Useful Properties of the Trees, Plants, and Shrubs* by Francis Peyre Porcher, published in 1863. This book was used by Confederate physicians and housewives alike. It gave a description of the plant, where it grew, what part of it to use, how to prepare it for use, and the ailments treated.

Physicians during the Civil War knew little about infection. For every soldier who died in the Civil War, on both sides of the battleground, of battle wounds, two more died of disease and infection, including diarrhea and dysentery. There was no knowledge of the cause of disease and no concept of hygiene. Amputation rates were high. Doctors didn't know to wash their hands or sterilize instruments and equipment.

The forerunner to Porcher's book is the *Medical Flora, or, Manual of the Medical Botany of the United States of North America, Volume 1* written by C. S. Rafinesque and published in 1828. Volume 2 was published in 1841. Rafinesque (1783–1840) was born outside of Constantinople but immigrated to the United States. According to Matthew Wood, author of *Vitalism, The History of*

Herbalism, Homeopathy, and Flower Essences, Rafinesque became a professor at Transylvania University in Kentucky and is considered an important field botanist of North America: "Rafinesque was a skilled practitioner of herbal medicine who gathered information from Indian medicine men and pioneer doctors. His descriptions of medicinal uses were concise enough to inspire the confidence of his readers." Rafinesque's work influenced Porcher and later the Eclectic physicians. There is also no doubt in my mind that Porcher must have also gathered information on herbs that were commonly used by the poor whites and slaves. It seems unreasonable to assume less.

After the Civil War, the former plantation system turned into a tenant system with basically the same landowners. The new system offered no racial preference in its exploitation; both poor whites and freed slaves were now at the mercy of the landowners. Both groups became sharecroppers, farming the land and paying a percentage of the profits to the landowners. My maternal grandfather was a sharecropper and raised cotton and corn for the landowner. My whole family had to work the fields in order to "pay back" the landowner.

After the Civil War, a series of laws continually elevated the status of poor whites and reduced the rights of blacks. But these laws did not change the fact that poor whites and blacks continued to do the same work, live in the same types of cabins, use the same herbal remedies, and share many of the same social experiences. White field hands worked alongside black tenant farmers, ate the same diet, and worshiped the same God. Wealthy landowners used these facts to elevate tensions between the poor whites and blacks who were competing for the same local resources. This continues even today.

Other than in a few of the larger cities, the general infrastructure of the Deep South during this era focused on getting the cotton to market. Railroads often stopped at rather isolated locations, whistle stops, just to load cotton, with nary a town in sight. In the hillier and more mountainous regions of the South, Appalachia was isolated by the rough topography of the land. Here, coal mining and the search for minerals formed the basis of economic development. Regardless of the landscape, the South was poor and herbs were needed to help when folks couldn't afford a doctor.

The sharecropper or land tenant system, along with the isolation and marginalization of the South, nurtured Southern Folk Medicine in unique ways to continue crossing racial and economic lines.

North of the cotton fields, the coves and hollows of the Southern Appalachian Mountains provided a similar isolation from the progress of the modern world. The poor grew corn for moonshine or worked in coal mines, but the same basic class structure was in place. Wealthy whites owned the land, stores, mines, and factories, and the poor whites and blacks worked to make the owners richer. After the Civil War, poor whites, and to a lesser extent, poor blacks, moved back and forth between the highlands and the lowlands of the Appalachians. Today, these two areas of the South are still among the poorest regions of the country and continue to share a common culture. I would also include Arkansas, parts of Missouri, and the hill country of northern Texas in this common shared culture. In some ways, very little has changed other than that most of us have internet now.

The Great Depression, from the 1930s to mid-1940s, further plunged the already poor population of the South into deeper poverty. As a region, the South didn't begin to recover economically from the Civil War and the Great Depression until the second half of the twentieth century, and some areas of the South have not fully recovered to this day. In these areas, the poverty is so constant and severe that my paternal grandfather, Herman Light, was fond of saying, "They said there was a depression. But we couldn't tell the difference."

The Great Migration of African-Americans from the South to larger cities in the North began after World War I and continued into the 1960s. The Southern agricultural system had collapsed due to worldwide economic depression. In addition, more farmers were using tractors and other modern farming equipment, and there was less demand for field hands and agricultural workers. Cotton was no longer king. Competition for the few remaining jobs between African-Americans and poor whites was at an all-time high. African-Americans that moved North were seeking a better life away from economic constraint and Jim Crow laws. In industrial cities, jobs in factories offered the opportunity for better education, less prejudice, legal rights, less violence, and economic advancement. Cities that saw massive influx include Detroit, Chicago, New York City, Philadelphia, and Pittsburgh. As opportunities in northern cities diminished, African-Americans moved west to Phoenix, Los Angeles, San Francisco, Seattle, Portland, and Oakland. This migration saw the spread of Southern herbalism to other parts of the country.

Not only were African-Americans moving from the rural South to the industrial North, but they were also moving from the rural areas to the bigger cities of the South, such as Atlanta, Birmingham, Memphis, and Houston. In whatever city they moved, their home remedies based on Southern Folk Medicine went with them. They were often willing to share their healing information to those in need or the curious.

For example, one of my beloved herbal heroes is James Duke, Ph.D. from Birmingham, Alabama. He worked for the United States Department of Agriculture (USDA) from 1968 to 1995 in the Agricultural Research Service as a botanist, and was the leader of the USDA Cancer Screening Laboratory. Dr. Duke developed a comprehensive Phytochemical and Ethnobotanical Database that is still used in critical research by scientists today. He is the author of more thirty books and hundreds of articles, written not only for the scientist and researcher, but also for the layman. I'm always curious when I meet another fellow Alabamian who is interested in herbs, so I asked Dr. Duke what sparked his interest. He replied, "When I was growing up in Birmingham, our African-American neighbor down the street was an herbalist. He let me follow him around pestering him with questions all day long, and I absorbed this like a sponge."

❧ FIVE ❧

Church, Superstitions, and Signs

*And God said, "Behold, I have given you every herb yielding
seed, which is upon the face of all the earth, and every tree,
in which is the fruit of a tree yielding seed; to you it shall be
for food."*

—*Exodus*

MY FEVER WAS SO HIGH that Mama said I was talking out of my head, not
making any sense at all. After I'd been sick for more than a week with fever,
lung congestion, and a cough and home remedies not working, Granddaddy
Light told my Daddy, "Enough of this. You get that girl to the doctor." So Daddy
loaded me into the truck for a doctor's visit, something rare at that time period
in our house. I was diagnosed with double pneumonia and a hospital stay was
recommended. In a time before health insurance, the family couldn't afford that
kind of medical care. So the doctor sent me home with antibiotics and a stern
advisement that if I wasn't better by morning or if my fever worsened during the
night, then get me to the hospital or I might die.

Back at home, the fever continued to rage and consume my body. It climbed
higher and higher and nothing seemed to bring it down. I coughed up green
mucus from my lungs in ever-increasing amounts until the effort was just too
great. Every breath became a raspy effort. Then, quietly and suddenly, I stopped
coughing and stopped moving. It was then Mama got on the phone and started
calling folks to come and pray for me. And they came.

We lived in a tiny house; the largest bedroom was barely large enough for a double bed and a dresser, and the living room was so small only a couch and a couple of straight chairs fit in. When I came to my senses, when I woke from the state of semi-consciousness in which I had fallen, all I could see from my bed was a sea of heads bowed in prayer. Folks from church had crowded into the room and were on their knees in prayer. There were people praying in the adjacent rooms as well. All was quiet except for the sound of many voices in prayer, each prayer individual but all rising and falling, creating a type of syncopation. The preacher reached down and picked up a bottle of olive oil and anointed my head while he spoke in tongue. After the anointment, the rising and falling of prayers lessened and folks, one by one, lifted from their knees and left the room.

Mama came and felt my forehead with her hand. "Praise the Lord," she said. My fever was gone and I was thirsty, and for the first time in days, I seemed to be able to think clearly. At that point I knew I was going to be just fine, but it was only later that I understood how close I had come to dying. My body still had to recover from the ravages of the fever and my lungs from the effects of the infection, but I was out of the danger zone. I had lost ten pounds in a very short time of illness, weight I could barely afford to lose since I was already too skinny. But there was no doubt in my mind that I was alive through Grace.

This wasn't the only time that church members were called to our house to pray for someone in poor health. Whenever the need was present, they were only a phone call away. And just as often, we went to another member's house so that Mama could help pray for someone else in need.

Mama was a Free Holiness, sometimes unflatteringly called a Holy Roller. Going to church was "going to meeting" and was a central part of our life. As a family, we attended meeting on Wednesday nights, Saturday nights, Sunday mornings, and Sunday nights and, of course, any revivals. Our social life revolved around church. The children we played with were either cousins or children of church members. These were the folks who showed up for funerals, wedding showers, baby showers, and during times of illness. Other than relatives, these were the people we depended upon. Several years ago, when Mama was nearing death, it was church members that brought food for us to eat so we didn't have to worry about feeding ourselves and could take better care of Mama. It was church members who took her to the doctor when we couldn't, and it was church members who stayed and offered support after her funeral. I still stay in touch with folks that I went to church with in my youth even though I haven't attended that church since I was a teenager. I still love those people.

When I was a child, my favorite part of meeting was singing. There was no formal choir because every person in church sang; we were the choir. We sang old-time gospel songs at the top of our lungs with complete abandonment—not hymns, mind you, but pat your feet gospel songs complete with four-part harmonies. After singing three or four songs, the preacher might say a few words, not generally a lengthy sermon, and members were then invited to stand and testify—to share with the congregation something about their lives that was bothering them, or how they felt blessed by God, or if they felt any conflict with another member. Sometimes when someone testified, the power of God struck and they moved across the floor under the power, almost a dance. Sometimes, under the power, they would be called to lay hands on someone else who might be in need of healing or cheering up, or on a sinner as a calling to repent.

After everyone who felt the call to testify had done so, another song or two was sang and alter call was announced so that any sinners who felt the call could come before the congregation and pray upon their knees for forgiveness of their sins. A person received the Holy Ghost and was forgiven of their sins when they completely and absolutely gave their life to God and spoke in tongue as evidence of this. If the members had confidence and conviction that this had happened, the person was accepted into the fold. Some folks spoke in tongue the first time at alter, others took years, and some strived but never achieved it. Once a person received the Holy Ghost, they could never sin again and still be part of church. Each person who received the Holy Ghost became a brother or a sister and prefaced other church members with that title. When I was growing up, Brother Morgan was the preacher and his wife was Sister Lettie.

When a person received the Holy Ghost, they were baptized, generally at a river or pond. The folks on the bank sang several songs (we did like singing), and then the person getting baptized would walk out into the water with the preacher. The preacher would put one hand on the upper back of the person and drop them back into the water and raise them quickly back up. Songs began again. Usually the freshly dipped person had dry clothes ready for a quick change behind a bush or car, and then we'd all go to someone's house for potluck. This was an opportunity for play with other kids, great food, and, sometimes, homemade ice cream. It was indeed a celebration.

Often, after Sunday service, we would be invited to go home and eat with another family. Sometimes we invited folks to come to our house after church on Sunday instead. Mama preferred cooking food and taking a covered dish to other members' homes because we didn't have indoor plumbing and guests had to use the outhouse. We were that poor.

Free Holiness kept themselves apart from general society as much as possible, preferring their community of fellow churchgoers. This has changed somewhat over the years as Southern society has changed and women have entered the workforce in ever-increasing numbers. Church women can't cut their hair, wear makeup, wear pants or shorts, smoke cigarettes, use profanity, or drink alcohol. Their hair is long and so are their dresses. Men can't have facial hair, drink alcohol, gamble, use profanity, and are pacifists in times of war. Men are the head of the household.

Men sit on one side of the church, women on the other, the kids somewhere in the middle, and sinners in the back. Free Holiness churches did not pay their preacher, though a collection was taken for building upkeep and to pay the travel expenses of guest preachers. To the day she passed, Mama wouldn't go to a church if the preacher was paid. She believed that preachers were called by God and no money should enter into that spiritual contract.

On the fourth Saturday night of each month was the Lord's Supper and footwashing. Only members who had received the Holy Ghost could participate. Unleavened bread was cut into small bite-size pieces and washed down with a bit of grape juice. After a few songs, two benches were turned to face each other on both the men's and women's sides of the church house. Songs began and continued through the whole process, literally for an hour or more. Basins were filled with water, and while folks were singing, every brother and sister washed and dried another's feet and had their feet washed and dried in return. Everyone sang and hugged, and the feeling of love and acceptance in the church was just amazing.

Free Holiness services are not dry and staid or filled with placid ritual. All church members participate—testifying to other members on God's influence in their lives and moving their bodies as the Holy Ghost calls them to move and speaking in tongue when graced. Services were filled with enthusiastic singing to foot patting gospel songs such as "I'll Fly Away" or "I'll Meet You in the Morning." All this shouting, singing, and praying created a unique spiritual energy that was a far cry from the sedate hymns and boring sermons of my school friends' churches. Free Holiness members understand the power of the spirit, recognize spiritual power in others, and expect that power to be used in Godly ways. The Holy Ghost could possess a person and fill their body and act as a conduit for healing energy by the laying on of hands. Voices lifted in song could be heard rolling across the land, inviting everyone to experience the joy of salvation. This common ecstatic spiritual experience brought folks together in a strong and supportive community.

Christianity

The principles and practices of Southern Folk Medicine can be used within any spiritual system, but I hope you appreciate the role Christianity played in its creation. This must be acknowledged and respected. Catholic missionaries came with the Spanish and immediately worked to convert the Native population. The Irish, Scots, and Scotch-Irish were Christians, either Catholics or Protestants, and other immigrating groups also brought the Cross to the New World. Both Native Americans and African slaves were soon indoctrinated with the Christian religious beliefs held by the growing and strong white culture, which would soon dominate the land and the peoples of the region.

Let's begin with the Spanish and the first recorded religious interactions with natives. In 1528, Panfilo de Narvaez, after having been blown off course in the Gulf of Mexico, landed at Florida instead of Mexico. This changed the lives of Native Americans in the New World forever. The Narváez Entrada made its way through Florida and into Georgia, Alabama, Mississippi, and Louisiana, exploring and mapping the land while searching for "Apalachen," where it was believed that gold and grain could be found in abundance.

From a journal of the time by Alvar Nunez Cabeza de Vaca, a member of the party: "We inquired of the Indians (by signs) whence they had obtained these things and they gave us to understand that, very far from there, was a province called Apalachen in which there was much gold. They also signified to us that in that province we would find everything we held in esteem. They said that in Apalachen there was plenty."

The governor, Narvaez, had been conned. Indian tales of gold in Apalachen were a trick to get him to move on and leave them unharmed. Along the way, in the search for Apalachen, many of his men and African slaves died from illness and injury, and others fled into the surrounding land hoping to survive with the local natives. "Most of the horsemen began to leave in secret, hoping thus to save themselves, forsaking the Governor and the sick, who were helpless," writes Cabeza de Vaca.

To facilitate the exploration of the countryside and to save the governor's life, the expedition was divided between land and sea. The ships, carrying the governor, sailed onward to Mexico with the expectation of a rendezvous with the remaining men who undertook an overland journey. This strategic mistake cost the Spanish. Disease, lack of food, unfriendly natives, and a foolish attempt to reach Cuba on rafts devastated the overland expedition, reducing the original crew of about 250 to four. The rafts landed not in Cuba, but off the shore of what is now Galveston, Texas. The four surviving original crew members were Cabeza de Vaca, Alonso del Castillo Maldonado, and Andres Dorantes de Carranza, and the African slave, Estevan, the first historical black man in America (also called Stephen the Moor and Black Stephen). It is from Cabeza de Vaca's journal that we gain knowledge of this expedition.

Castillo, Carranza, Estevan, and Cabeza de Vaca lived for several months as the slaves of various Indian tribes, helping gather firewood, water, and wild foodstuffs. Prickly pears were an important survival food for the group, and the narrative contains numerous accounts of the gathering of this fruit along with others, as well as edible roots. Upon escaping their tenure as slaves, the castaways' fortune changed for the better when they were accepted as free men by the Avavares tribe in South Texas. Improving their position even more, the castaways became adept at healing prayer. Tales of their abilities grew and preceded them upon their journey.

From Cabeza de Vaca's journal: "The very night we arrived, some Indians came to Castillo telling him that their heads hurt a great deal, and begging him to cure them. After he made the sign of the cross on them and commended them to God, they immediately said that all their pain was gone. They went to their lodges and brought many prickly pears and a piece of venison, which we did not recognize. Since news of this spread among them, many other sick people came to him that night to be healed. Each one brought a piece of venison and we had so much we did not know where to put the meat." Cabeza de Vaca's journal entry cites the first documentation of faith healing in the New World.

The castaways became the rock star healers of the New World. Their fame spread across the land, and sick natives walked miles to receive the faith healing prayer; Castillo became the most accomplished and the most willing to take on extreme cases. Cabeza de Vaca writes: "When I neared their huts, I saw that the sick man whom we were supposed to heal was dead, because there were many people weeping around him and his lodge was dismantled, a sign that its owner was dead. When I got to the Indian, I saw that his eyes were turned. He had no pulse and it seemed to me that he showed all the signs of being dead. Dorantes said the same thing. I removed a mat that covered him, and as best I could I beseeched our Lord to be pleased to grant him health and to grant health to all who needed it. After I made the sign of the cross over him and breathed on him many times, they brought his bow to me along with a basketful of ground prickly pears. Then they took me to cure many others who had sleeping sickness....They said that the man who was dead and whom I had healed in their presence had gotten up well and walked and eaten and spoken to them, and that all the people we had healed had gotten well and were very happy. This caused great wonder and awe, and nothing else was spoken about in the entire land."

The castaways left the Avavares tribe and headed toward Mexico, hoping to meet up with other Christians. Along the way, natives brought their children to be blessed, the sick came to be healed, and for this service, they were well-fed, often given the tribe's best food. They received other gifts: bows and arrows, flint, precious stones, and hides.

Cabeza, the bold, performed the first surgery by Europeans in the New World in northern Mexico, when he opened the chest of a wounded warrior and removed an arrowhead lodged near the heart, then stitched the wound closed. The Spaniards continued their journey, winding their way back to Texas, returning to Mexico, and then heading toward the Pacific Coast, and always, the word of their healing abilities preceded them.

After eight years of living with various tribes, Cabeza de Vaca returned to Spain and finished the journal about his experiences in the New World in 1540. The journal became the talk of the town and even before its publication made Narvaez a hero. Cabeza's best-selling journal, *Relación*, was published in 1542 and urged a charitable policy toward the natives, one most Spanish ignored and one that was believed to later contribute to his fall from grace. Cabeza's journal, though initially written as a personal memoir and travel journal, provides a wealth of information for scholars and historians. In 1544, the government of Spain began legal proceedings against Cabeza for his visionary policies, and in 1551 he was banished to North Africa.

By the early 1500s, the first interactions between the Spanish, their African slaves and the Native Americans had already taken place. Healing, herbal, food, religious, and survival information was being exchanged in a way that would forever change all cultures concerned.

The Bible

It is not the scope of this writing to delve into all the interactions of early Christians and the Native peoples or African slaves. The focus here is to acknowledge that interactions did take place and to acknowledge the role of Christianity in the early development of Southern Folk Medicine. This would be incomplete without mentioning the importance of the Bible itself.

The family Bible was often the only book the settlers and poor people owned. It was, and still is for many Christians, a reference book for daily living and a guide to good health. The family Bible held records of family marriages, births, and deaths, and in lieu of governmental agencies held legal and binding records. When Mama was in her early sixties, she discovered that a birth certificate or proof of birth was required to apply for Social Security. She had been born at home and, at that time, there was no legal requirement to register a birth. In order to establish proof of birth, Mama used the family Bible along with notarized statements from relatives who were alive when she was born. She felt quite an achievement when her birth certificate came in the mail.

The family Bible and the Blue Back Speller were often used to teach reading to homeschool students. Children were needed to work on the farms and that meant forgoing proper schooling. Schools could also be miles from where folks lived, and children had to walk or be taken by wagon.

The King James Version of the Bible is the English translation completed in the early 1600s and approved by the Church of England. Being translated in that time period means that it is filled with humoral language. For my Mama, the King James Version was the *only* official version of the Bible, and she admonished me more than once not to read any other.

The Bible itself is sometimes used as a healing tool. For example, it can be opened to a specific passage relevant to a situation and placed under the bed for four days and nights. This is thought to help those who are sick to effect change in their lives that will lead to healing. A Bible can be placed under the bed to keep away bad dreams. A Bible either under or by the bed can be a source of comfort and companionship. Opening the Bible and believing that a certain scripture is an answer to a question or offers direction is considered a form of divination and was very popular in the Appalachian Mountains. It's also thought that sleeping with a closed Bible under the pillow will allow you to dream the answer to your problem.

Customs such as this made their way from the British Isles to Appalachia and the Deep South. For example, Elizabeth Mary Wright remarks in *Rustic Speech and Folk-lore* that to find a husband, "after supper, then wash up the supper dishes and go to bed without speaking a word, placing the Bible under your pillow with a pin stuck through the verse previously read; or place a Bible under your pillow with a crooked sixpence over the verses: 'And Ruth said, Intreat me not to leave thee, or return from following after thee....'" Quotations and passages from the Bible were also used to support a principle for healthy healing or the use of herbs or essential oils for health or for spiritual cleansing.

Herbs in the Bible

The Lord hath created medicines out of the earth; and he that is wise will not abhor them.

—Ecclesiasticus 38:4

Herbs are mentioned throughout the Bible, both as remedies and for spiritual cleansing. Because they were mentioned in the Bible, some people believe these plants have extraordinary healing powers. There are 128 plants mentioned which were used for food, cosmetics, medicine, and religious ritual. Some herbs, especially shrubs and trees, were made into essential oils.

Many of the herbs and foods mentioned in the Bible were native or able to grow in Israel, and some were introduced through trade. I'm not going to discuss all 128 plants mentioned in the Bible, but I will mention a few that continue to be used today. This is also a validation of the safe and effective use of many herbs which have a history of thousands of years of use. Talk about empirical evidence!

Aloes were used to heal skin irritations and burns and to embalm the dead. To avoid confusion, scholars believe that the aloes mentioned in the Bible are not the cactus variety, *Agave americana,* found in the New World, but rather the *Aloes agallocha* tree. This tree produces a fragrant resin and a high-quality wood of which the heartwood was the most prized for its resin. That being said, minus the fragrance, the aloe tree and the aloe cactus are used for many disorders, including healing burns, sunburn, and skin irritations. Aloe has an affinity for the skin and soothes and protects damaged skin.

It is said that the pharaohs fed *garlic* to the slaves to keep them strong and healthy while they worked on the pyramids. Whether this is truth or legend remains to be seen, but garlic helps build a strong immune system, helps lower cholesterol, and helps lower blood pressure. Used topically, garlic is anti-infective and antimicrobial. Garlic has an affinity for the lungs and is traditionally used for asthma, bronchitis, and pneumonia. And, it helps ward off evil spirits and vampires. How awesome is that? I could talk for an hour on garlic, it has such amazing health benefits, but space prohibits this.

It is generally accepted that the *anise* referred to in the Bible is actually *dill;* both plants have similar healing properties, though opposite tastes. True anise is slightly sweet with an underpinning of bitter. True dill is slightly sour with an underpinning of bitter. Both are aromatic plants whose main healing properties are found in their essential oils, which come from the seeds. Both are plants of the Mediterranean area, and both help soothe irritated bowels, and are useful for colic and indigestion and gentle enough for babies. Other properties or uses of both plants include to aid diuretic activity, as an expectorant, to increase milk flow, to ease menstrual pain and cramps, as a sleep aid, and as an aid to stop smoking.

Bay or *bay laurel* or *sweetbay* is one of my favorite herbs. Traditionally, bay laurel represents wealth and prosperity. The Greeks and Romans made crowns of laurel to adorn the head of victors of athletic events and military campaigns. The head of Apollo is depicted adorned with a wreath of bay laurel. It's also used to denote a graduate of higher learning and used in some commencement exercises. King David had his personal rooms paneled in bay laurel, and today the leaves in emblems decorate many churches and temples.

The dried leaves of bay are used in soups, stews, and in vegetable and meat dishes. It's used as pickling spice, and its antioxidant activity reduces food spoilage.

Bay is a digestive aid, increases the flow of bile, and reduces intestinal gas. It has antifungal and antibacterial properties, and, I do believe, immune-stimulating properties. Bay has also traditionally been used to lower blood sugar. It has been used topically for skin cancers, infected hair follicles, and for dandruff. This herb is in one of my favorite formulas to boost the immune system and one that personally works for me. If I feel that I'm coming down with a virus and take this formula immediately, it usually reduces the amount of time I'm sick if not stopping it altogether. This is based on a Dr. Shook formula and includes pine bark, bay, cayenne, and cloves.

These are just a few of the herbs listed in the Bible that are still being used today similarly to their traditional uses. I can't think of a better testimony to the safe and effective use of these herbs.

The Signs

> Let there be light in the firmament of the heaven to divide the day from the night; and let them be for signs, and for seasons, and for days, and years.
>
> —Genesis 1:14

That was the Bible verse most often quoted to me by my mother-in-law, a staunch believer in the Signs, who also went to church at least three times a week. The Signs, also called the Man of Signs or Almanac Man, were used to plant the garden, harvest produce, cut hair, bale hay, set important dates, potty train the baby, find the best days for hunting and fishing, and just about anything else. I was a young adult before I realized that this was actually astrology—folk astrology

As an oral tradition, folk astrology, based on sun and moon signs, has survived in the South and Midwest longer than other parts of the United States and Europe. It's not complex astrology. As a matter of fact, most of the people who practice folk astrology depend on an almanac for vital information, such as the constellations where the sun and moon are located on any given day. The solar zodiac is divided into twelve signs (constellations), and the sun stays in each sign about thirty days. On the other hand, the moon moves fast across the sky and rotates through the twelve constellations about every two-and-a-half days. In folk astrology, it is the moon that is most important.

The use of the almanac is a tradition that clearly made its way from the British Isles and Europe to the United States. An early documentation on using moon signs along with the pictorial representation of man dates back to 1496, in *Margarita Philosophica* by Gregor Reisch, published at Heidelberg. This is the forerunner of the Almanac Man that became highly popular in the original colonies.

Early almanacs contained all sorts of useful information. Here is some advice from the British *Husbandman's Practice or Prognostication Forever* (1664): "Good to purge with electuaries, the moon in Cancer; with pills, the moon in Pisces; with potions, the moon in Virgo. Good to take vomits, the moon being in Taurus, Virgo, or the latter part of Sagittarius; to purge the head by sneezing, the moon being in Cancer, Leo, or Virgo; to stop fluxes and rheums, the moon being in Taurus, Virgo, or Capricorn; to bathe when the moon is in Libra, Aquarius, or Pisces; to cut the hair off the head or beard when the moon is in Libra, Sagittarius, Aquarius, or Pisces." While all this is interesting information, the part I find most fascinating is that bathing was only recommended four times a year. Things had to have gotten pretty smelly in between.

In colonial America, *Poor Richard's Almanac* (1732–1758), published by Benjamin Franklin (writing as Richard Saunders), was full of wit and wisdom and a wealth of information based on astrology. Franklin's almanac was a combination of puzzles, herbal remedies, witty sayings, proverbs, verses, humor, and weather predictions (based on astrology). An early form of the Man of the Signs appeared in the 1741 issue—a man is seated on a globe surrounded by the twelve signs in a square. The current form of the Man of the Signs, standing with limbs outstretched and surrounded by symbols, appeared in *Poor Richard, Improved*, in 1783.

As commonly drawn for the last fifty years, the Man of Signs stands naked with outstretched arms and legs. In some drawings, his bowels are exposed, but in others they are not. Lines are drawn from twelve different body parts to symbols around the body. The origin of this concept began in ancient Babylonia and was further developed by the Greeks. Christian mystics adopted the concept of "signs in the heavens," and it gained much traction with medieval astrologers and became a popular concept. Nicholas Culpeper (1616–1654) wrote a most complete application of the concept in *Astrological Judgement of Diseases from the Decumbiture of the Sick* (1655), which is also a treasure drove of herbal information. According to Culpeper, "There is a sympathy between Celestiall and Terestriall bodyes which will easily appear if we consider that the whole creation is one entire and united body, composed by the power of an Allwise God of a composition of discords. Also there is friendship and hatred between one sign of the zodiac and another, for fiery signs are contrary to watry and nocturnall to diurnall, etc."

Almanac Man or the Man of Signs divides the body into regions, beginning at the head and working down to the feet. Each region is governed or influenced by an astrological sign. Here's the basic breakdown found in the almanac; a more in-depth version is often used by herbalists and health astrologers.

Head—Aries, which rules fevers, inflammation, sinus problems, metabolism, and muscular strength and speed.

Neck—Taurus rules the thyroid, sugar metabolism, beauty of hair, skin, and eyes, and lymph nodes.

Arms—Gemini rules the lungs, trachea, bronchial tubes, arms, hands, shoulders, fingers, and the sympathetic nervous system.

Breasts—Cancer rules the chest, breasts, stomach, esophagus, diaphragm, and the left side of the body.

Heart—Leo rules the heart, upper back, spine, spinal cord, and the thymus gland.

Abdomen—Virgo rules the intestines, solar plexus, and abdomen, as well as the parasympathetic nervous system.

Reins—Libra rules the kidneys, adrenal glands, skin, and the lower back.

Secrets—Scorpio rules the bladder, urethra, reproductive system, colon, and sweat glands.

Thighs—Sagittarius rules the hips and thighs, the sciatic nerve, and the liver.

Knees—Capricorn rules the bones, joints, and connective tissue, as well as the knees, hair, nails, and teeth.

Legs—Aquarius rules the blood circulation and the internal oxidation process, the calves and ankles, and the valves of the heart.

Feet—Pisces rules diseases that are difficult to diagnose or cure, the feet and toes, as well as the spleen and the lymphatic system.

Catfish Grey, an Appalachian herb doctor from West Virginia, used folk astrology to understand certain kinds of illnesses. Catfish believed that, based on astrology, people are susceptible to "two-way viruses" (colds, flu, measles, mumps, chickenpox) in cycles. Every twenty-eight days a person's astrological sign "comes due," and that person will be particularly susceptible to an infection for a period of about two days (the time the moon stays in a sign).

Different parts of the body can also be more vulnerable to injury depending on a person's sign. For example, a Sagittarius might be more prone to hip or thigh injury when the moon is in the sign of the thighs (Sagittarius). To continue the analogy, when the moon is in the corresponding sign, an Aries might be more susceptible to head colds, headaches, and sinus infections; a Libra to kidney infections or cystitis; a Pisces to swelling in the feet; an Aquarius to tight calf muscles and nerve pain; and a Leo to heart palpitations.

The signs are also used for the planting and harvesting of crops. In general, fire and air signs are barren—Gemini, Leo, and Virgo are the most barren, followed by Aries, Sagittarius, and Aquarius. Earth and water are considered the most fertile signs—Cancer, Scorpio, and Pisces are considered the most fruitful, followed by Libra, Taurus, and Capricorn. This is generalized and there are exceptions. For instance, the earth sign Virgo is considered barren, while the air sign Libra is considered fruitful.

Some general advice for the planter: Never plant on the first day of the new moon or when the moon is changing quarters. Plant above-ground crops in the first quarter, plant crops that vine or grow close to the ground in the second quarter, and plant root crops in the third quarter. Plant above-ground crops in the waxing or growing moon and below-ground crops in the waning or decreasing moon.

Folk astrology is alive and well, and there seems to be a renewed interest in planting by the signs. *The Old Farmer's Almanac,* which has been in continuous publication since 1818, sells about four million copies each year and is often quoted in my area, especially the weather predictions. I'll close this chapter with a quote from a song by Randy Travis, "The Family Bible and the Farmer's Almanac," writing about his grandfather and the two books he believed in most: "Words to live and die by front to back, the family Bible and the farmer's almanac."

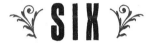

SIX

Tenets of Southern Folk Medicine

For in the true nature of things, if we rightly consider, every green tree is far more glorious than if it were made of gold and silver.

—*Martin Luther*

IT WAS THE giant white oak that drew her to that particular acre of land. It was a family tree with branches spreading wide across the yard, a huge trunk reaching toward the sky. Huge roots pushed above the ground and then plunged deep within the Earth. It was the tree that first attracted her to the piece of land but there was also a well.

There had once been a house next to the well, but the youngest child of the previous owners had fallen in and drowned, and then the house caught on fire and burned to the ground. They just didn't have the heart to rebuild and so had moved on, leaving the land to return to pasture and weeds, except, of course, for the massive oak. There was another tree on the property, a hickory, but it was half rotten and slightly leaning. But it was the oak tree that drew her, and that's how Mama found the land. She knew about the child dying in the well, but that didn't stop her from wanting the acre as she didn't consider herself the superstitious sort. The well water was clean, there was plenty of room to build a house, and there was a huge garden spot with rich soil for planting. And then, there was the tree.

So, she worked hard in the cotton fields saving her money. She hoed, chopped, weeded, and thinned the cotton. And later in the fall, when the boles were wide-open and white as snow, she picked and pulled until her gloves were shredded and her hands were too. She managed to save every penny from her hard, sweaty work. She saved $500 cash, enough to buy the piece of land. A whole acre—she was now a landowner.

With an acre homestead outright owned, Mama then had the collateral to purchase a Jim Walter home, a shell house. The Jim Walter company completed the outside of the home watertight but left it up to the customer to finish the inside themselves. No corners were straight and the ceilings were low, no plumbing, no electricity, and no inside walls except for studs, but it provided a dry place to live in the meantime. This was the state of the construction when we moved in. She wouldn't fully complete the house until many years later when all the children were grown and gone from home. There wouldn't be enough money until then.

The oak tree is massive, a giant among trees, a Family Tree. At the smallest part of the lower trunk, the tree measures nineteen feet around. The branches reach across 116 feet of the front yard, providing shade to the house and across the road on the other side. We didn't have the luxury of air conditioning, but under its canopy we shelled peas, shucked corn, ate meals, cooled off, held family reunions, hosted visitors, and watched the traffic go by. It was an extension of the house, and the yard under the tree was kept as neat as any other room with extensive mowing and raking.

The lower branches are so wide that you can walk across them, but a ladder is required to even reach the first branch. Much of my childhood was spent under that tree playing games, reading, riding my bike, working, and sometimes just being. I wrapped my arms across the trunk and cried when my father died, pouring my grief and sadness into its stout form. I sat on its exposed roots, leaned back against the trunk and told the tale of my divorce to a nonjudgmental and willing ear. I've felt the depth of its roots and the beating of its core, its heartwood, and I couldn't tell the difference in our heartbeats. I've slept at its base and entered the doorway of another world. And the tree took it all.

It is the center of the world, a perfectly shaped Tree of Life, beautifully illustrating the connection between the Underworld and Heaven. It is clearly a symbol of earth and air. It is the tree that stood in the garden, its leaves for the healing of the nations. It is a symbol of resurrection, losing its leaves in the fall as the sap moves to the core and sprouting them anew in the spring as the sap rises and moves outward. In Southern Folk Medicine, our bodies are like the tree. In the winter, our blood thickens and moves inward to our core, keeping the vital organs warm and protected. And in the spring, our blood thins and moves outward, bringing life back to our extremities, just as the sap rises to the branches.

A host of indigenous peoples have legends of the Tree of Life. In Ireland, every clan had a mother tree, an oak, under which chieftains were appointed and gatherings were held. The Celts believed that the soul of every person was tied to the soul of a tree. The Romans, and later the Catholic Church, destroyed many oak groves on the British Isles because they were sacred to the Druids. African legends hold that the first man and woman were carved from a tree. The Cherokee built the sacred fire from oak, and burning twigs were offered to each direction. And who can forget that Tolkien's Ents, man-like tree herders, symbolize the talking trees found in many cultures around the world.

In Appalachia, a tree was often planted at the birth of a child; this was known as the birth tree. The tree and the child were linked, and as long as the tree was healthy, the person stayed healthy. The clothes of a sickly child could be hung on a stout tree to make the child better, and, in this way, some of the tree's strength was imparted to the sick one. Sometimes rags were tied to these trees and they were considered spiritual places where magic could still be found. And there were also bottle trees, so named because bottles were tied upside-down to tree branches to catch evil spirits.

My family tree has many, many branches. Hundreds at least. My sister Brenda is the historian who has followed these branches from one country to the next. Some branches are as strong as the trunk of a tree and some are much smaller, reflecting continued growth in a new direction. I like to think of those branches as bits and pieces of our lives as a family. From my Daddy and his branches, I learned about the herbs and plants in the woods, how to read animal tracks, how to watch for snakes, how to throw a knife, how to read the Signs, how to let wild things be wild, and how to wander. And I am ever grateful for the traditional healing knowledge that he and my grandparents carried across the generations.

From my Mama, I learned about hard work, how to keep a clean house, how to raise a garden and preserve food, how to take care of kids, how to read dreams, how to tame wild things, how to pray, and the importance of roots. She loved that piece of land with all her heart and didn't leave it until the day she died.

We are the seeds that carry forth. We embody the gifts, thoughts, and history of those who came before us, and we will pass the information to the branches that come after. Within us is the sap of generations of people who lived and loved and passed on their knowledge and traditions in ways that we may not comprehend at the moment, but which become clearer with time. So let your branches grow stronger, lift your leaves to the heavens, and stand rooted in your beliefs.

The Tenets of Southern Folk Medicine

According to the Merriam-Webster dictionary, a tenet is a principle, belief, or doctrine generally held to be true; especially: one held in common by members of an organization, movement, or profession. Basically, as pertaining to Southern Folk Medicine, the tenets are the principles upon which the practices are based. Please keep in mind that this is a metaphorical language, but that does not in any way detract from its truth.

1. Fluids move around the body like the sap in a tree.

In Southern and Appalachian Folk Medicine, the body is likened to a tree, and fluids move around the body like the sap in a tree. In the cold of the winter when the days get shorter, the sap falls and moves from the peripheral limbs to the branches and down into the trunk. Likewise, in the human body, the blood vessels constrict and blood flow to the surface of the skin is restricted. The constriction shifts circulatory patterns from the capillaries to the arterioles. This increases the work of the heart and will raise the resting pulse. As the weather gets increasingly colder, blood flow is restricted to the peripheral limbs and pulls inward to protect the core of the body and to warm the vital organs. The reduction in blood volume may also increase blood pressure, causing high blood until the body adjusts. The body tries to compensate by increasing fluid loss with increased urination, which is why you want to pee when you get really cold. As the weather gets even colder, the body will alternately constrict and expand the capillaries to the skin's surface to keep it healthy while maintaining a core temperature until the season change.

As the days get longer and the weather gets warmer, the sap rises, moving up the trunk to the limbs, then to the branches and young twigs. Likewise, in the human body, the blood moves outward from the arterioles into the capillaries, reinvigorating and awakening the body. At the same time, the vessels dilate and increase blood flow to the surface of the skin in order to disperse heat. Initially, the dilation will cause low blood, but as the heart works harder to manage the increased circulation required to disperse heat, high blood may result in a rise in pressure. You may have experienced this feeling by getting so hot that you feel the pulse throbbing in your temples. The blood is high, the body is working hard to disperse the heat, and the throbbing in your head is warning for you to slow down and cool off. Sometimes a person will experience low blood during the day and high blood at night as the temperature changes from hot to less hot. In the spring, the pulse moves toward the surface and has a more wiry feel. It is important to stay hydrated to reduce strain on the heart.

In the winter, the goal is to keep the vital internal organs protected and warm and the brain active. In the summer, it's the opposite. The goal is to keep the vital organs and the brain cool and functioning at peak efficiency. If the temperature is too cold, it's hard to think. If the temperature is too hot, it's hard to think. In hot weather, the blood must disperse the heat from the internal organs and keep the vital organs cool. The head increases sweating and heat loss to keep the brain cool. In the heat of the summer, the pulse is on the surface and very strong. In hot weather, dehydration can also increase heat and increase pulse, and cause heat stroke, sun sickness, and stroke.

Impurities or pathogens the body has been harboring over the winter can rise with the coming of the spring. Summer or fall illnesses can be contained over the winter when the blood is thick and then "come up" or manifest in the spring when the blood begins to move again. Spring cleansing of the body is an important aspect of Southern Folk Medicine, helping thin the blood and get it ready for summer and helping remove any pathogens or impurities that have over-wintered.

Blood-purifying spring tonics include sassafras tea, red clover, prickly ash, yellow dock, plantain, burdock, chickweed, yellow root, Oregon grape root, sarsaparilla, echinacea, garlic, young poke greens, and various herbal laxatives.

Like leaves on the trees, which change their angle to the sun and sweat to keep cool, we humans must do the same. As long as you are sweating, body heat is dispersing. The dangerous situation occurs when the sweating mechanism shuts off.

2. Observation of the fluids of the body and their movement provide a measurement of the state of the health of body.

The important fluids of the body are blood, lymph, mucus, bile, sweat, tears, and feces. These are the fluids excreted from the body that are the most observable. You cut yourself and you bleed. You eliminate urine and feces. You scrape your skin and it weeps lymph. You vomit and vomit until there is nothing but bile. You get a cold and blow out mucus. The observation of these fluids in Southern Folk Medicine is obviously due to the influence of the Greek humoral system so prevalent in Europe, the Middle East, and North Africa at the time of the settlement of the New World.

These fluids and their movement around the body are critical for health. While the state of the blood is considered the most obvious and important indicator of health in Southern Folk Medicine, as it is in modern medicine, the other fluids are also important. Let's take a quick look at each of them.

Blood is the river of life. It supplies essential substances and nutrients, such as glucose, oxygen, infection fighters, and hormones to our cells. It then carries waste such as carbon dioxide, urea, and lactic acid away from those cells. Eventually, this waste is released from the body through the organs of elimination as urine, feces, sweat, and carbon dioxide. It's a pretty simple but effective method. Blood also helps regulate our body temperature. During strenuous exercise, very warm weather, physically demanding work, or fever, there is increased blood flow to the surface of the skin. The skin feels warm, may turn red, and there is faster heat loss. When the climate turns cold, the blood flow shifts in order to protect the important organs deep inside the body.

Herbs that move the blood include American ginseng, black cohosh, cayenne, red root, hawthorn, safflower, peach leaf, blueberry or huckleberry leaves, willow bark, red clover, fenugreek, prickly ash, and garlic.

Herbs that build the blood include American ginseng, angelica, nettles, red clover, alfalfa, yellow dock, beets, kelp, fennel, and sarsaparilla.

Herbs that reduce the flow of blood include yarrow, cayenne, shepherd's purse, wild geranium, plantain, goldenseal, yellow root, aloe vera, and calendula.

Lymph is the clear liquid that oozes from the skin with a carpet burn or scrape. Its primary function is to carry infection-fighting substances, white blood cells, to the site of injury or invasion. The lymph system helps rid the body of toxins, waste, and other undesirable matter. While the blood circulates in a continuous loop—away from and to the heart—the lymph only flows in one direction, toward the heart. The blood has the heart to pump it around the body, but there is no lymph pump. The lymph depends on muscle movement such as walking, deep breathing, and exercise for circulation. This makes it extremely important that you move and exercise for good immune functioning.

Herbs that move the lymph include bayberry, blue vervain, black walnut, blue flag, cayenne, chickweed, cleavers, echinacea, fennel, fenugreek, fringetree, mullein, poke, red root, stillingia, violet, bear's-foot, and wild indigo.

Mucus is the result of the irritation of mucous membrane tissues—sinus passages, bronchial tubes, lungs, esophagus, stomach, gallbladder, small intestines, large colon, kidney bladder, urethra, ureters, and female reproductive tissue of the uterus, fallopian tubes, and vaginal canal. As you can see, most of our internal organ systems are mucous membrane tissues, excluding the liver and kidneys. The mucous membrane tissues protect the organs and systems that interact with the outside air or external environment. When irritated, mucous membrane tissues excrete mucus to capture and isolate the offending substance; whether pollen, bacteria, viruses, or semen, so the body can eliminate it. the body can eliminate it. Mucous membrane tissue protects the stomach from stomach acid. It protects the bladder from the irritation of urine. It protects the gallbladder from the irritation of bile. Hardened mucus is called canker, and a number of herbal remedies soften canker so it can be removed. Mucus can be clear, cloudy, yellow, or green. Most folks have observed this color change during a cold or sinus infection. These color changes can sometimes be observed in the stool or in the coughed-up mucus due to a lung irritation or infection.

Herbs that move mucus include mullein, elecampane, fennel, lobelia, pleurisy root, red root, slippery elm, sweetgum, marshmallow, plantain, wild cherry, white pine, wild plum, and horehound.

Herbs that reduce the flow of mucus include goldenseal, yellow root, barberry, bayberry, hyssop, mountain mint, peppermint, rabbit tobacco, sage, red raspberry, sweetbay magnolia, and fenugreek.

Herbs that soften hardened mucus include anise, fennel, sarsaparilla, sweetgum, mullein, chickweed, violet, hydrangea, mimosa, boiled okra water, and Solomon's seal.

Bile is secreted by the liver and stored in the gallbladder, where it is released during a meal. The main purpose of bile is to break down or emulsify fats with detergent-like action. It also contains waste from red–blood cell breakdown, known as bilirubin, which is dumped in the gastrointestinal tract to be eliminated from the body if enough fiber is present. Bile also contains cholesterol, water, minerals, and metals, which are also released into the gastrointestinal tract for elimination. Even though it's called bile acid or bile salts, bile is actually alkaline, not acidic. In addition, and most importantly, bile takes away waste produced by the liver from the breakdown or metabolism of toxins and pharmaceuticals.

Herbs that stimulate the release of bile include yellow dock, barberry, goldenseal, American ginseng, milk thistle, blessed thistle, gentian, dandelion, and almost any bitter herb.

Sweat is moisture that is released through the skin due to heat, fever, exertion, or emotional distress and fear. It contains, first and foremost, salt. During the hot summer temperatures, construction workers and others working outdoors must be cautious to take in enough salt and water to prevent dehydration. I've seen the t-shirts of construction workers with white rivers of salt after a full day of work. Sweat, like urine, also contains urea, ammonia, and sugars. Although sweat may carry a trace amount of toxins, the main detoxifiers of the body are the liver and kidneys. Women generally don't sweat as much as men even when exerting the same amount of energy, which may be due to circulating hormones.

Herbs that increase circulation and induce sweating are generally given as hot teas. These include blessed thistle, boneset, butcher's broom, cayenne, elderflower, hyssop, mugwort, red root, sarsaparilla, sweetbay magnolia, and yarrow. Cayenne, black pepper, ginger, and horseradish can be added to foods to increase the heat and induce sweating.

Tears help keep the eyeball clean and wash away irritating substances. What cook hasn't experienced tears when chopping onions? Like sweat, tears contain salt, with the addition of some protein, water, mucus, and oil. Tears are produced continuously at a low level to keep our eyes lubricated. Tears are also produced due to stress, anger, grief, or other strong emotions. These emotionally induced tears also contain stress hormones, prolactin, and other hormones to enhance mood.

Herbs that can help moisten the eyes include hydrangea, eyebright, bilberry, blueberry, fennel, and evening primrose oil.

BODY FLUIDS

Our body fluids are divided into two important divisions: intracellular fluids and the extracellular matrix. All fluids inside the cell are known as intracellular fluids and contain a high level of potassium. The extracellular matrix comprises all the fluids outside the cell and generally contains high levels of sodium. The exchange of sodium and potassium or extra- and intracellular fluids creates the charge of electricity that sends signals throughout our nervous system.

Each of the humors or fluids looks different, smells different, and tastes different. The condition of the fluids—color, odor, viscosity, texture—can be an indicator of an imbalance in the body, an organ system functioning less than normal, an infection, or fever. Southern Folk Medicine is concerned with the information inherent in the condition of the fluids. For the Greeks, a cause of disease could be the surplus or deficiency of a humor; in Southern Folk Medicine, the surplus or deficiency of a fluid is an indicator or symptom of a health problem, not the problem itself. We will look at each of these humors or fluids in greater depth when discussing the constitutions and elements.

3. Measurements of humors or fluids such as blood, urine, and mucus, are described as pairs of opposites.

Many measurements or assessments used in Southern Folk Medicine are in pairs of opposites. Most likely this is based on the Pythagorean Theory of Opposites, which was used in the Greek system of healing. Pythagoras (570–495 BCE) was a famous philosopher who stated that in order to understand something, you have to have experienced its opposite. To understand one, you have to understand the many. To experience the finite, you have to understand the infinite, and so on.

Another Greek philosopher, Heraclitus of Ephesus (535–475 BCE) also contributed to the same theory. He believed that everything had an opposite, and when these two opposites were in harmony, there was peace. He also believed that opposite tensions resulted in harmony. It is in the opposites that we become aware. Being close to death makes us appreciate life. Being sick makes us appreciate good health. And being hungry makes us appreciate our food.

When changes occur to one pair of the opposites, then problems occur in the other.

4. Good health is achieved when our opposites are in balance and we are not exhibiting any excess or deficiency symptoms in our body or personality.

If you think about the concept of excess and deficiency of our health on an imaginary scale, with deficiency being too little (1) and excess as too much (10), there are all the numbers between 1 and 10 that might describe our health. Balance, or being "just right," is achieved somewhere around the number 5. It's an arbitrary scaling system to be sure, but I think it adequately illustrates the concept.

5. The state of the blood is a measurement of the state of the body. Blood measurements or qualities are high/low; good/bad; fast/slow; thick/thin; and hot/cold.

In Southern Folk Medicine, the state of the blood is described in pairs of opposites: high/low, good/bad, fast/slow, strong/weak, thick/thin, and hot/cold. We can extend the pairs of opposites to reading the pulse: tense/relaxed, even/choppy, and wide/narrow. I refer you to the book *Traditional Western Herbalism and Pulse Evaluation: A Conversation* by Matthew Wood, Francis Bonaldo, and Phyllis Light (2015) for further reading on the pulse based on Southern Folk Medicine's concept of opposites. But now, let's look at the most common pairs of opposites of the blood characteristics.

High blood may refer to high blood pressure or blood congested in the upper part of the body above the heart. This is often seen in folks who are overweight and who are alcoholics and diabetics. It can be evidenced by a red face and broken vessels around or on the nose. High blood can cause pounding headaches, blurry vision, watery eyes, ringing in the ears, drowsiness, nausea, dizziness, blacking out, and chest pains. At the extreme, high blood can cause stroke, heart attack, shortness of breath, and lethargy. The blood may also be sweet and thick, with elevated pressure.

Herbs and foods to thin the blood, get it moving, and lower the pressure are helpful. My favorite herbs for high blood are cayenne, blue vervain, garlic, American ginseng, Queen Anne's lace, black cohosh, valerian, and hawthorn berries.

Low blood can be defined as the position of blood in the body (congested below the heart), low blood pressure, or anemia. Blood congested in the lower part of the body tends to occur around the feet and ankles as evidenced by broken vessels in those areas, stagnation in the female reproductive system, and congestion in the small intestines. Low blood may cause memory loss and poor thinking ability. Low blood sugar and dehydration may also play a role. Other patterns of low blood include fatigue, tiredness, low spirits, lack of will or drive, stroke, dizziness upon standing, blacking out, weakness, constipation, lassitude, paleness, cold hands, feet, or limbs, thinness or low body weight, dry skin, pale fingernails, cracks on the heels, rash on the lower legs or feet, and dry, listless, or thinning hair. Folks with low blood also tend to exhibit a lack of will, drive, or motivation. Low blood may also strain the heart. Herbs and foods to build the blood are helpful.

My favorite herbs for low blood, a deficiency state, are yellow dock, burdock, sarsaparilla, red clover, alfalfa, American ginseng, fennel, peppermint, black cohosh, saw palmetto, nettle, angelica, and chlorophyll. Nutrient-dense foods are also needed, such as beets, dark green leafy vegetables, beans, and animal protein.

Good blood refers to a person in a state of good health. A person with good blood has energy, vitality, and a creative spark or an active mind. The skin is clear and so are the eyes. The emotions are balanced and there is good mental health. Good blood can also refer to genetic inheritance or "good genes."

Bad blood refers to an unhealthy state of the body, a chronic illness, a parasite infection, or a sexually transmitted disease such as syphilis.

The term *bad blood* was so commonly understood in the South that in 1932, the Public Health Service began a study to record the progression of syphilis among infected African-American males in Tuskegee, Alabama—the "Tuskegee Study of Untreated Syphilis in the Negro Male." According to the Centers for Disease Control and Prevention (CDC), "The study was conducted without the benefit of patients' informed consent. Researchers told the men they were being treated for 'bad blood,' a local term used to describe several ailments, including syphilis, anemia, and fatigue. In truth, they did not receive the proper treatment needed to cure their illness. In exchange for taking part in the study, the men received free medical exams, free meals, and burial insurance. Although originally projected to last six months, the study actually went on for *forty years [emphasis mine]*." Yes, you are reading correctly: forty years. What horror for the men and their families. Even when penicillin was shown to be a treatment for syphilis in 1947, it was not offered to participants in the study. In 1972, the study was discontinued as unethical. Talk about bad blood....

Bad blood can also refer to an association of emotions such as anger, hostility, or bitterness. In the Appalachians, bad blood might happen between families as a result of an argument or insult. Feuding families might talk about bad blood between them. Participants in the Tuskegee Study might experience feelings of bad blood with the government.

Bad blood can also refer to poor genetics or "bad genes." Folks with inherited bad blood might exhibit a birth defect, cross-eyes, withered arm, cleft palate, or mental illness. Bad blood might also be a sign of intermarriage between cousins or other close relatives.

Herbs that support the organs that clean the blood are known as alteratives or blood cleansers, and include: echinacea, goldenseal, yellow dock, prickly ash, red clover, chickweed, sarsaparilla, sassafras, dandelion, Oregon grape root, poke root, plantain, violet, garlic, blue flag, blessed thistle, St. John's wort, cleavers, cascara sagrada, common buckthorn, senna, turkey rhubarb, butternut, and wahoo.

Herbs to treat or remove parasites include: black walnut, Queen Anne's lace, male fern, wormseed leaves, pink root, hyssop, pomegranate root, pumpkin seeds, papaya, rue, garlic, nigella, cloves, mugwort, myrrh, onion, quassia, thyme, and wormwood.

Fast blood and *slow blood* refer to the movement of blood around the body. This can often be felt in the pulse. A racing pulse can denote fast blood. Folks with fast blood may have heart palpitations, sweat easily and often, and have trouble sleeping. There may be endocrine imbalances such as thyroid issues or very reactive adrenal action. Folks with fast blood may exhibit temper, impatience, be very energetic, and talk a lot.

Herbs to help slow down fast blood include most nervines, but my favorites are: passionflower, valerian, lemon balm, lemon verbena, spearmint, bugleweed, blue vervain, motherwort, wood betony, black cohosh, and hops.

A slack pulse can denote slow blood. Folks with slow blood may exhibit lethargy, fatigue, slow thinking, and brain fog. There is a definite lack of motivation and drive. Folks rest and sleep as much as possible and are often quiet within themselves and prefer being away from crowds. The body may be cool and feel damp to the touch. Slow blood is often found in chronic illness, thyroid issues, inflammatory disorders, and bad or dirty blood disorders. Slow blood may also be deficient or low and need building, as in the case of anemia.

Herbs for slow blood include kelp, cayenne, red clover, and peppermint, along with all the herbs mentioned under bad blood to cleanse and low blood to build. This should be undertaken in stages—build first and then cleanse. Never cleanse a person in a deficiency situation; it only creates more deficiency. Sometimes building the body is needed before cleansing.

Thin blood is watery and slow to coagulate. Though thin blood is not always considered to be low, it can lead to low or weak blood. Summer's heat and alcohol thin the blood. Thin blood is pale and light red in color, lacks substance, and has little or no texture. There may be a lack of iron in the blood, and anemia may be associated with thin, weak blood. Stress, severe illness, and nerves can also contribute to thin blood. A person with thin blood appears pale, sunken-eyed or has dark-circles around the eyes, is wane, tired, and listless, and lacks backbone or courage. Many of the patterns associated with thin blood are the same as those associated with low blood. This is a deficiency state, and building herbs may be needed.

Herbs to address thin blood are also the same herbs used to address low blood. Foods to address thin blood are dark green leafy vegetables, beans, beets, and animal protein.

Thick blood coagulates quickly, is dark red, and has a gummy texture. Thick blood is considered dry and moves slowly around the body. It may be high in iron. Thick, dry blood is often associated with high blood pressure or "stuck" blood. A person with thick blood tends to be lethargic, moves slowly, and gains weight easily. Urine will tend to have the same characteristics as the blood, being thick, dry, and dark yellow. A person with thick blood may also have sweet blood or diabetes, along with high blood pressure or cardio-vascular disease.

Herbs for thick blood include: cayenne, American ginseng, feverfew, garlic, ginger, turmeric, dong quai, peppermint, red clover, chamomile, bilberry, black cohosh, motherwort, and St. John's wort. Supplements that thin the blood are fish oil, vitamin E, vitamin A, quinine, cinnamon, oregano, papain enzymes, bromelain, and the foods blueberries, grapes, pineapple, and papaya.

Hot blood can be the result of diet, season, environment, sexual desire, acid blood, fever, inflammation, or illness. The most common form of hot blood is fever. The person with hot blood may also have skin eruptions or rashes, hives, increased sexual drive, or frazzled nerves. A person with hot blood may present with heart palpitations, be underweight, and wiggle. Fluids and watery fruits can help cool down the blood. A person with hot blood should avoid hot baths or showers.

Herbs to cool down hot blood include yarrow, elderflower, peppermint, boneset, chamomile, blessed thistle, Monarda, sage, catnip, spearmint, hydrangea, marshmallow, and yucca.

Cold blood can be the result of extended or chronic illness, a damp, cool environment, wind, sudden temperature change, not enough sex, or too many cool foods. Cold produces mucus which is harbored in the body, especially in the lungs, bronchi, bladder, stomach, gallbladder, and digestive tract. Mucus may harden in any of these areas, causing further damage. A person with cold blood is sluggish, tired, has stiff joints, and inflammation of the muscles may also be present. Certain disorders such as low thyroid, fibromyalgia, or chronic fatigue may result in cold blood. Because the blood is cold and lacks digestive capacity, nutritional status is low.

Herbs to warm the body include cayenne, milk thistle, American ginseng, blessed thistle, red clover, black pepper, peppermint, cinnamon, cloves, angelica, kelp, licorice, sarsaparilla, and sassafras.

6. The four properties are hot/cold and wet/dry. This applies to the body, foods, herbs, medicine, the climate, relationships, and most anything else in life.

The concepts of hot/cold and wet/dry are so important that I've devoted a whole chapter to them. Please see Chapter 7 for a complete discussion.

7. Blood Tastes, known as Southern Blood Types, are used to describe the constitution of a person: bitter/salty; sweet/sour.

Blood types may be in excess, deficiency, or balance. These will be discussed in greater detail, along with specific herbs, for each constitution in the next chapter. Here's a brief summary of excess or out of balance of each type.

Bitter blood is often thin, weak, and watery, with low pressure. Stagnation is often found in the digestive tract, and leaky gut syndrome, yeast overgrowth, or parasites may be present. This results in incomplete emptying of the bowel and the accumulation of wastes in the gut that hijacks the immune system. People with bitter blood may appear bloated, have a pale face and thin, pale fingernails. Nutritional status is low. There can be a tendency toward heart palpitations, coldness over various parts of the body, dental problems, and stooped shoulders and back. They may be holding a hurtful grudge or be obsessing about a past event that they just can't let go. A person with bitter blood has little drive or creative fire; all their fire is going to thinking about the past. They tend to isolate emotionally and think about whatever past event has negatively impacted their life, whether a divorce or a lost job. Herbs and foods that strengthen digestion and move blood and lymph are helpful.

Salty blood is weak and wet. Moisture is high, and there may be fluid retention in the hands, feet, and face. A person with excess salty blood tends to look a bit bloated all over. Salty blood is often found in women going through menopause, those with hypothyroidism, and people who are chronically ill, have autoimmune disorders, or have liver or kidney disease. The salty person tends to feel victimized and seeks sympathy from others. Helping the excess salty person enjoy activities and people is an important step in balancing their blood. Drying herbs and foods are helpful if not taken in excess.

Sour or acid blood is somewhat thin and bright red. It is associated with heat in the blood, summer's heat, and inflammation in the body. Persons with excess sour blood may exhibit rashes, red spots, and food and chemical sensitivities. They may be prone to food allergies and should avoid acidic foods such as citrus fruits, tomatoes, sugar, red meat, and breads. Excess sour blood folks may have anxiety or panic attacks, as well as test and sports anxiety. These folks like to debate and argue and will often take the opposite stance in an argument even if they don't agree with it. Herbs and foods to sweeten the blood are helpful. Most necessary is addressing fears and insecurities.

Sweet blood is thick and syrupy, and creates an environment for parasites. In excess sweet blood, there is a tendency toward diabetes and high blood pressure. These folks are often overweight or obese, have a red face, and exhibit shortness of breath. Body fat tends to be centered around the abdomen, with large belly and small or stringy arms and legs. A self-centered personality sets the stage for overindulgence or addiction. A person with sweet blood may have a tendency toward self-importance and tendency to be a packrat. Sweet blood may also be thick and high.

8. *The four elements are fire, earth, air, and water.*

Remember that the language of folk medicine is built on metaphor and allegory. Folks know that the four elements aren't actually the elements in the periodic table. They are elements of composition and believed to be essential to life. The four elements will be discussed in greater detail in the chapter on constitutions. Here's a brief summary of the characteristics of each.

Fire is the great catalyst. It transforms, changes, or consumes all that it touches. Fire spreads across the land, jumps here and there, or smolders. This is true whether it's the fire of digestion, the fire of the thyroid, or the fire of emotions. Fire people are creative, passionate, and extroverted, and make good leaders. Temper and anger emerge when they are under stress.

Water follows the path of least resistance across the land and in the body. It can slowly wear away mountains and carve valleys. Water can be a trickle or a tsunami. It always flows downward with the lay of the land and gravity. Water people are relationship-oriented, creative, and intuitive. Tears emerge under stress.

Air moves across the land carrying dust, rain, and electrical signals. Blowing wind can wear away a mountain, stir up a dust devil, or cool the fevered brow. Air can be still, a slight breeze, or a strong gale. Folks with strong air are intelligent, have sensitive nerves, and love the idea of things. Hurtful words emerge under stress.

Earth is the mother of us all. It is solid, strong, and stable. There are several different types of earth: sand, clay, loam, chalk, peat, and silt, each with its own characteristics and fertility. Earth people are practical, hard-working, and security-oriented. They like to design, build, and grow. Quietness emerges under stress.

9. *There are three types of illnesses: physical, psychological, and unnatural or spiritual.*

Physical illnesses are often acute in origin, such as bacterial or viral invasion, parasites, or injury. They may also be associated with stages of life, such as childhood illnesses, problems associated with growth spurts, fertility issues, menopause issues, and health problems associated with aging.

Chronic illnesses are physical disorders that have a strong mental/emotional aspect. These include autoimmune disorders, lifestyle-oriented disorders such as diabetes, disorders resulting from exposure to environmental toxins, trauma, chronic stress, and post-traumatic stress disorders. The longevity of the illness wears away at the Vital Energy and can create depression and a sense of hope-lessness of healing, which makes it even harder to make decisions or to do the very lifestyle changes that are needed to improve.

Psychological or mental/emotional health issues include mental health issues, addiction, depression, a case of nerves, mental disturbances, and nervous breakdown. Sometimes, the first sign of a chronic illness is a personality change. Any time there is a huge personality change, look for either a physical illness, such as infection, or a nutrient deficiency.

Unnatural or supernatural illnesses require additional expertise, such as from those trained in roots or faith healing, or someone trained in counseling. In the old days, this would have included hexes and possession, but today would include chemical imbalance. Causes of this imbalance are addiction, acting out due to sexual abuse, or intense feelings of guilt or fear.

10. We are made of the clay of the Earth, so when we get sick, we must go to the clay (minerals) for our healing.

What is the clay of the Earth? Clay is a combination of minerals in the ground and, according to scientists from Cornell University, acts as a breeding labora-tory for tiny molecules and chemicals which it "absorbs like a sponge." From the Bible to Native American cosmology to Chinese mythology, legends say that humans were made from the clay of the Earth. Although the clay itself may seem infertile, in Earth's early history, it was far from that. Clay and water form a hydrogel that soaks up chemicals from its surroundings, providing a protective home for developing proteins.

The human body is made of the same basic minerals as the Earth. However, we can't just crush a rock and expect to absorb the minerals from it. Plants are the intermediary between the minerals in the Earth and the human body. They absorb the minerals, process them into a useable form, and then we consume the plants.

In Southern Folk Medicine, we must return to the clay for our healing. Plants that reach the clay of the Earth include all trees, plants with long taproots, and plants that push through the Earth, breaking it apart.

Some of my favorite herbs that reach the clay of the Earth include: black walnut, magnolia, dogwood, yellow poplar, sweetgum, tag alder, elderberry, sumac, cedar, juniper, slippery elm, hawthorn, witch hazel, mulberry, grapes, pine, cramp bark, red clover, wild grapes, mullein, alfalfa, burdock, yellow dock, and dandelion.

11. We are part of the Earth and cannot separate ourselves from it.

We are made from the clay of the Earth and are as much a part of the Earth as the rocks and the trees. There is no spaceship to save us when we have overpopulated and overpolluted the Earth and it will no longer support life as we know it. The Earth is the mothership, providing food, water, and air for all life, and we are dependent upon it. There is no way around that fact.

Our body's defense system, our immune system and organs of elimination, works hard to keep us healthy in an onslaught of pollen, bacteria, and viruses. What happens when we add a slew of pollutants or toxins to the list? This creates a body burden, a total accumulation of pesticides, toxins, herbicides, metals, petroleum byproducts, and other pollutants that can affect health over a lifetime. It's the accumulation over a lifetime that's the issue, not the occasional light exposure.

We can't separate ourselves from the Earth. It's God's supreme creation made just for us. Some folks just don't appreciate the gift.

12. God made the plants before we were made; plants are here for our food and medicine.

The plants evolved and populated the Earth before either animals or humans. From a practical point of view, let's consider that both humans and animals breath oxygen. It's a fact that oxygen is only produced as a byproduct of photosynthesis, which is how plants create food and energy from sunlight. Algae, kelp, phytoplankton, cyanobacteria, trees, shrubs, and grasses make all the oxygen on planet Earth. So you see, green came first to create the oxygen environment for humans and animals.

The plants also provide food, timber for building materials, herbs, rubber, fuel, dyes, perfumes, natural pesticides, natural fibers for clothing, and prescription medications. Over 25 percent of medications contain plant isolates, and a huge number of synthetic drugs were developed from plants. We are dependent upon the bounty of plants for our very existence.

13. For every illness there is a specific plant.

Both Native American cosmology and Bible verses support this tenet. The issue then becomes, how do you find that right plant? How do we know a plant is the right one to use? With attention to constitutional assessment, listening to the person's story, a good understanding of human physiology and patterns of dysfunction, and a working knowledge of the properties and uses of plants—that's how we do it.

Since every person is different, the remedy that works for one person in a given situation may not work for another person. It's not as simple as one herb for one pathogen, which is the hallmark of the conventional medical approach. The bacteria, viruses, and single-cell eukaryotes that reside within us—the microbiome—are essential for human life and outnumber human cells about ten to one. To be healthy humans, we must nourish our microbiome with foods and herbs, not kill it off with prescription medications (unless absolutely needed).

14. The plant/herb you need is always growing close by or where you need it, or is a sign of something that needs attention.

Sometimes, the herb a person needs is growing right in their backyard or is a sign that it is needed. Dandelion is my favorite example of this. Of course, this is a very common yard herb and one that landscape companies strive continually to remove from those perfect lawns. When I pass a house whose front yard is just full of dandelions, I wonder about the health of the inhabitants. Are they on multiple medications? Is there great anger in the house? Do they excessively drink alcohol? Are their livers under stress? I passed a house the other day and the front yard was just full of thistle. I wondered what kind of prickly situation was going on in that house.

15. The antidote grows next to the poison.

This is often true of the wild plants. Poison ivy and its antidotes are a good example of this. Many herbalists are familiar with plantain or jewel weed as poison ivy remedies, but there are others. Tommie Bass recommended boiling plantain in milk for poison ivy. Other favorite herbs applied as washes include white oak bark, pine bark, witch hazel, or any astringent herb. You'll often see poison ivy climbing an oak tree or a pine.

I was once leading an herb walk and stepped off the path to talk about an herb at the edge of the woods. Unknowingly, I had stepped into a bed of poison ivy while wearing a dress and sandals. After I stepped back on the path and resumed the walk, a student walked up to me and whispered in my ear that I had been walking and standing in poison ivy for about five minutes. Going back to the site, I noticed plantain growing along the edges of the path also. I grabbed handfuls of plantain, squashed it good, and rubbed it up and down my lower legs and feet. Nary an outbreak or rash did I have.

16. Bitter herbs have the strongest medicine.

There are four tastes in Southern Folk Medicine: bitter, salty, sour, and sweet. Of all the tastes, bitter herbs are considered to be the strongest, based in part on the fact that they taste so bad. "If it tastes bad, it must be good for you," is an old expression. Even Mary Poppins sang, "A little bit of sugar makes the medicine go down."

Foods and herbs taste bitter due to alkaloids, lignans, and other phytochemicals. The plant develops these secondary metabolites for protection against bacteria, fungus, viruses, and parasites, and we get their benefit when use them. The bitter taste also helps protect us against spoiled foods and poisons. Our natural reflex with extremely bitter foods is to spit it out.

17. Good digestion is the basis of good health.

Eating is a life-giving process that should be nourishing for the mind, body, and spirit, and shouldn't cause any difficulty with properly prepared foods and a healthy digestive tract. We tend to take eating for granted, cramming the activity into busy schedules without taking the time to rest and digest after a meal. That's one reason why so many Americans suffer from some type of digestive difficulty such as bloating, gas, abdominal pain, or inflammation.

From beginning to end, the digestive tract is about twenty-eight to thirty feet long, the small intestine is about twenty-one to twenty-three feet long, and the large intestine is about five to six feet long. But the digestive tract is more than just the colon. It includes the mouth, esophagus, anus and rectum, and auxiliary organs: the liver, gallbladder, pancreas, tongue, salivary glands, and teeth.

The purpose of digestion is to transfer nutrients, water, and electrolytes from food to our internal environment. In the process, we convert fats and carbohydrates into useable or storable forms of energy. Protein is converted into base amino acids and used to build muscle, repair tissue, and make neurotransmitters, blood components, or enzymes. The process of digestion converts vitamins and minerals into useable, absorbable nutrients.

Keeping the digestive tract healthy and avoiding disorders such as stomach ulcers, leaky gut syndrome, irritable bowel syndrome, or autoimmune disorders should be a priority for everyone. The digestive tract is in direct contact with the outside world or the external environment. You eat something and it immediately begins interacting with the digestive system. The food that you eat has an immediate bearing on your health and state of mind.

"You get what you pay for" is an old saying that has major application when we buy food. If you buy cheap food that is high in calories and devoid of nutrients, then chances are that over time your digestion will begin to suffer for this, and so will your health. First there is discomfort and bloating, then more bloating, belching, pain, cramps, constipation, and/or diarrhea, until finally the digestive system is overwhelmed and disorder or disease results.

Digestion and immunity are directly linked. The human digestion system houses about 70 percent of the lymphatic system. That's huge—just think about that for a moment. The digestive tract is a primary entry point for bacteria into our bodies on a daily basis and must always be on guard. The small intestine houses the majority of the gut-associated lymphoid tissue (GALT) in the digestive tract. If our gut immune system is continually under attack from food chemicals and additives and high bacteria counts in food, then our body's immune system has been hijacked and isn't available for fighting off a cold, warding off an infection from a cut, or killing a cancer cell. So you see, the healthier our digestive tract, the healthier our immune systems.

We are back to the microbiome again. In order to keep our digestive system healthy, we must ensure that we have a healthy ratio of good to bad bacteria in our gut. For about every one human cell, there are about ten bacteria that aren't us, aren't human. The majority of these, minus a few bad bacteria or freeloaders, are necessary for life. To nourish our microbiome we should limit antibiotics and eat foods that nurture our good bacteria. Fermented foods are an excellent choice to support gut health, and supplemental probiotics can be taken when needed.

Regular bowel movements are necessary to eliminate the toxins which would normally leave the body through this route. If we don't have normal, daily bowel movements, those toxins and irritants have a field day wreaking havoc on delicate mucous membrane tissues, leading to inflammation, digestive difficulties, possible bleeding, and polyps in the large colon. You have to keep it moving. Drinking at the very least sixty-four ounces of water daily is important to help lubricate the bowels. Eating cooked foods, such as dried beans, greens, and vegetables, and some raw fruits is important to provide the necessary fiber requirement. Healthy cooking oils are vital, and the quantity should be defined based on your constitution. And finally, exercise and move. If your body is stagnant, then your colon is stagnant.

18. Chronic disease starts in the gut.

Hippocrates said, "All diseases begin in the gut." Obviously, not all diseases start in the gut, but many do. This wouldn't apply to genetic illness, certain bacterial or viral infections, parasites, or exposure to toxins. However, when we take into account that the gut houses a whopping 70 percent of the immune system, it's easy to see how this affects our general immunity and immune response, regardless of the cause of the illness.

Gut health affects immune activity, plain and simple. Sometimes a person's first inkling of a physical problem is digestive discomfort. Viewed in isolation, digestive problems may simply be due to overeating or poor restaurant choices. However, viewed holistically, when digestive problems turn into food sensitivities that turn into leaky gut syndrome that turns into ulcerative colitis, there is a huge issue. The red flag should have been waving around food sensitivities. Any change in digestion is a signal that something is not right. It's signaling that attention needs to be paid to overall health, not just digestive health, and to slow down and take time to figure out what's bothering digestion. A food elimination diet can be very helpful to determine any food sensitivities.

The very nature of a chronic disease or autoimmune disorder is that it slowly builds in the body. It can take about five years from the onset of symptoms until a problem can be accurately diagnosed by blood work.

Digestive problems can also lead to depression. Scientists have discovered that about 90 percent of our serotonin is produced in the gut by bacteria. Serotonin is a neurotransmitter that affects the nervous system, moods, muscle activity, and our sense of happiness and well-being. Drugs that affect serotonin are some of the most prescribed mood-enhancing drugs used in conventional medicine.

Bottom line: Gut health is a reflection of overall health and our sense of well-being. When in doubt, work on the gut.

19. Every person is born with a talent, and we must find and use our talents to grow who we are and become ourselves.

If we deny our talent, if we deny ourselves, this may cause unhappiness, depression, and illness. So what is a talent? In this context, a talent is any gift or leaning innate within us. It may be creative, such as art, music, or dance. You might be a natural-born athlete or love flower arranging or building things from wood. You might have an aptitude for business or chemistry. It may be an ability such as being a good listener or having an aptitude for foreign languages.

Even though we may have been born with a talent or leaning, it still takes practice, practice, practice to become skillful and expert with the talent. All the innate talent for music, athletics, or math may lie dormant or not reach full potential without study and practice. Manifesting your talent isn't about achieving greatness, becoming famous, or becoming rich. It's about fulfilling that bit inside you that yearns to express that which is waiting.

More than likely, this tenet made its way into Southern and Appalachian Folk Medicine from the Bible. There are several Bible verses concerning talents. The most commonly quoted one is from 1 Corinthians 12:7-11, which basically says that gifts (talents) are given for the common good. One person may have the gift of wisdom and another the gift of knowledge. Other gifts mentioned are for healing, languages, prophecy, and teaching.

20. Faith healers can lay on hands, talk out fire, bloodstop, or talk off warts.

These are all gifts that may be apparent at birth but more commonly are given from one person to another. These folk traditions can be found in the South and Southern Appalachians, the Ozarks, the Midwest, around the Great Lakes area, and really all across the country.

Touch therapies for healing are found in almost every culture and folk medicine in the world. They are extensively documented in the traditional medicines of China, Tibet, Egypt, Japan, and India, and among Native Americans and African Folk Healers. To touch someone who is ill is an automatic response and provides comfort, reduces anxiety, and soothes the nerves. Mothers touch and hug their children when they are ill or injured. And often all it takes for the child to feel better is a kiss from Mom. Modern laying-on-of-hands methods include Reiki, Therapeutic Touch, and reflexology.

Laying on of hands is referenced in both the Old and New Testaments of the Bible and is used in religious and healing ceremonies within a religious context. In this setting, laying on of hands transfers the healing power of God to the person in need who may be too sick, tired, or ill to pray themselves.

Talking out fire and bloodstopping are skills that can be passed from one person to another. A woman can teach a man these skills and a man can teach a woman, but a woman can't teach a woman and a man can't teach another man. Once a person teaches another to either bloodstop or talk out fire, their own ability is lost. They've passed it on.

Reference to bloodstoppers appears in manuscripts from the eighth century in Britain, Scandinavia, and Germany. A Bible verse is quoted under the breath while the bloodstopper holds one hand over the head of the person who is bleeding.

Fire-blowing takes away the pain of a burn, though it can also be used for any type of pain. Traditional Native American spiritual healing may involve sucking out the pain or blowing out the fire (pain). Blowing and sucking away pain have been documented among Native American tribes from the East Coast to the West Coast of the United States. Instead of blowing out the fire, I was taught to suck it out and spit it onto the ground. This is called drawing out the fire.

In some areas of Appalachia and the Midwest, fire-blowing may be called "talking out the fire." The fire-blower murmurs a Bible verse while holding a hand over the affected area.

There are probably more home remedies for warts than the common cold. Many of the home remedies, such as soaking the affected area in vinegar, using the herb thuja, or crushing an aspirin and applying as a paste, may have some scientific basis. But the more colorful wart remedies, which seem to work just as often as anything else, have no basis in science, such as rubbing a penny around the wart three times and throwing away the penny; tying a thread around the wart, leaving it overnight, and then burying it in a graveyard the next day; and rubbing the wart with a slice of potato and then burying the slice.

Locally, Cousin Calvin was considered the best wart-talker. People came from far and wide to have him talk off their warts. Calvin would wave his hand over the affected area, mumble a few undecipherable words, and tell the person that their wart would be gone in a few days. Warts disappeared fast enough on folks that Calvin developed a solid reputation that stood the test of time. I once asked Calvin what he mumbled, to which he replied, "Whatever takes my fancy for that person." He didn't have a set verse but tailored each individually. Another time I asked, "How does this work Calvin? What makes the warts disappear?" To which Calvin replied, "It's my energy. My energy has to be stronger than the wart and people believe this to be true."

21. Cleanliness is next to Godliness.

Although this is often attributed to the Bible, this phrase is not actually found within its pages. The source is most likely the Jewish Talmud. In 1605, Francis Bacon wrote, "Cleanness of body was ever deemed to proceed from a due reverence to God." John Wesley, the founder of the Methodist church, said in one of his sermons in 1791, "Cleanliness is indeed next to Godliness."

Whatever the source, cleanliness is an important concept in Southern Folk Medicine. From a practical point of view, an unclean house can harbor bacteria, fungus, and mold and mildew, and be a home for small critters such as rats, fleas, scabies, or lice. In older times, it was important to keep the house as clean as possible because folks lived very close to the elements and to nature, and there was often very little barrier between indoors and outdoors.

A clean house and a person who bathed regularly and wore clean clothes were signs of a person with good character. A person who routinely had an unwashed body and wore dirty cloths was considered to have low character, was considered unclean. Or as my mother was fond of saying, "Nasty." She encouraged me to have cleanly dressed friends whose mothers kept clean houses.

The concept of clean and unclean didn't rely on social status. For several years Mama earned money for our family by cleaning houses for some of the better-off families in town. She understood that even though these folks had a tremendous amount of money in comparison to her, they weren't always clean people. And in her eyes, this greatly lowered her view of their character. She once told me, "When I leave their houses, I know I've made a difference in their lives because I've cleaned it up." And she was right.

Even though we were extremely poor, our house was so clean you could eat off the floor. (No joke.) When a house is untidy, the floors haven't been swept, nor the dishes washed, and clutter is everywhere, this effects the physical body, the mood, and the mind. The buildup of dust, dander, pet hairs, and dust mites can affect allergies and creates a haven for fleas and germs. The clutter also creates an environment where it's easy to lose things like car keys, shoes, and bills. How do you find what's missing in all that clutter? Just the overwhelming presence of clutter increases anxiety and stress, and makes you feel tired. If your surroundings get too cluttered, the thought of cleaning both becomes and feels like an overwhelming task. Even more importantly, all that clutter blocks anything new from entering your life and encourages holding on to the past.

22. At the deathbed, burn cedar, stop the clocks, and cover the mirrors. Place a coin, generally a penny, over the eyes.

Birth and death rituals are an important part of any folk medicine. Many of these rituals have lost their place in the community but traditionally were there for a reason. My elders suggested never taking your newborn into a public place or having visitors, other than family, until the baby was at least three months old, if not older. This was to protect the newborn with an immature immune system from catching whatever was going around. Words of wisdom to be sure.

While birth rituals were times of joy, death rituals were a time of grief and, in my family, more important than birth rituals. They were especially important to my Mama. During the deathbed vigil, small cedar branches were often burned to "clean the air." Cedar is a sacred herb for Native Americans of the Southeast, along with tobacco, white sage, and rabbit tobacco. Traditionally, burning cedar at the deathbed purified the spirit and sent it along the way; it also scented the air. Stopping all the clocks and watches was a way to record the moment of death. My aunt Sadie told me that covering the mirrors kept the spirit that was leaving from seeing their reflection, realizing they had died, and trying to go back into the body. A penny was placed on each eye to keep them shut, but also to pay the ferry to cross the River Jordan.

If a woman had passed, the women family members along with other women in the community would wash the body, fix the hair, and dress the body for burial while singing gospel songs. If a man had died, the male members of the family and male community members washed the body, dressed the man in his burial suit, and either shaved the man or combed his hair and beard. The women would sing gospel songs in the next room.

All this had to be completed fairly quickly while the body was somewhat pliable and before rigor mortis set in. Mama and Daddy were often called upon to help in this capacity. This was in the days when the body was kept at home for the wake and taken to the church for burial. It would be called a green burial today, but back then, it was what poor people did who couldn't afford a funeral home or a fancy funeral. It was important to Mama that we all had proper burials, and she took out burial policies on each of us.

Our house, as poor as we were, was often the home where the bodies of family members came for the wake. The coffin would take up any spare space in the living room and would be open day and night until the funeral. Family and folks in the community would come in and out over about two or three days, bringing food, "sitting up" with the corpse, and telling stories about the person's life. Generally, it was men who sat up at night, not the women. For me, it was a really spooky time to tip-toe past a corpse on my way to bed, and I was often scared of going to sleep, lest I be haunted. On the upside, neighbors and community members brought food to eat and their kids with them, and we could play outdoors. As children, we weren't shielded from death. It was the final act of life.

23. A person's story can help reveal their illness.

Even though I've listed this last, this tenet is one of the most important ones to me. Each of us has a story, and throughout this book I relate a few of mine. My mother and father, grandparents, children, lovers, husbands, clients, and friends have influenced my story in ways that I could never have imagined. Much of my formative family story centered around that acre of land with the giant tree.

We all have many stories; these are the stories that have shaped who we are and how we live our lives. And when we pass this Earth, what we leave behind is our story. Many of our stories develop from events in our lives, some good and some traumatic, and these are the ones that create our personal identity—how we see ourselves, how we view our world, and how we find our place in it. And these are the stories that make our personal narrative.

Some stories develop about us or around us, and of those stories, we may be unaware—these are the ones that create our public persona or myth. These are the stories that shape how others see us and see our place in the world. Family is really good at sharing stories about us, especially at holidays, although they are not always the ones we want to hear. It's also often very true that our families see a different story than our friends because our story is also part of their story. Due to this, they filter the story through their lens of experience, which may not be the same as ours.

Hearing and understanding a person's story is a great assessment tool. Often, living the same story over and over is at the root of chronic health problems. This may include dating the same type of person over and over, being in a relationship that is no longer rightful, or holding onto beliefs that no longer serve a purpose. A person's story can hold them immobile and impede their healing journey. Unhealthy beliefs may center around self-esteem, feelings of belonging or worthiness, or traumatic life events. Regardless, the event or belief becomes an element in our personal stories the moment they occur or we think them into being. They become us.

Sometimes, an illness actually becomes the main character in a person's story. This happens when a person loses the dream, the vision, of who they are and allows the image of others to take over. As a matter of fact, whenever we have a symptom, it immediately integrates into our story. Before we know it, the illness may have its own personality, causing behaviors to be exhibited that are not normal for our personality. This is because a new personality has been introduced into the story, and a new relationship has gained prominence.

In Southern Folk Medicine, discovering a person's story is half the assessment process. This is how important their story is to understand. It is their narrative, their life in words. Without the story, how do we truly know the full extent of the events that led up to their illness? Without the story, how do we know who they are? Without the story, our approach is allopathic. Without the story, we are not thinking in a holistic manner encompassing mind, body, emotions, and spirit—a basic tenant of folk medicines around the world. Everything centers around the story.

I encourage you to spend some time discovering your own story and working to change any aspects of the narrative that no longer serve a purpose in your life. It will free up tremendous amounts of energy and open the door to new stories.

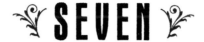

SEVEN

Hot/Cold and Wet/Dry

When clouds appear like towers, the earth is refreshed
by showers.

—*Old weather saying*

LIVING IN TORNADO ALLEY certainly offers a glimpse into the concept of hot/cold and wet/dry that many people rarely experience. A tornado happens when different temperatures and humidity meet. In the Southeastern United States, tornadoes form when warm, wet winds from the Gulf of Mexico meet the cold, dry air dropping down from Canada. Often, it seems like they are meeting right over my town, and in some ways, they are.

Hot and cold describe temperatures, and wet and dry describe humidity. Normally, warm air rises, which makes your attic the hottest spot in your house. When the hot from the Gulf meets the cold from Canada, the cold air traps the warm air beneath it. Perfect tornado weather. The warm air really wants to rise but can't, and so it begins to rotate in agitation. During the day, the sun continues to heat the ground and more warm air keeps trying to rise. This continues until the warm air creates enough rotation, agitation, and mass to push through the cold air holding it down. Now there is a flip-flop, and the risen warm air now traps the cold air beneath it. This creates the rotating column of raging wind and rain that is the tornado. One year, on February 14, it was 80°F during the day, and that evening after the tornado passed, it snowed.

There's no weather event more destructive than a tornado, which can reach speeds exceeding 200 miles per hour. Tornadoes happen more frequently than hurricanes, and cause more damage in the local area. Hurricanes reach speeds between 70 and 100 miles per hour, and tend to cause more destruction with flooding. In tornadoes, I've seen pine needles stuck horizontally into trees; pieces of hay embedded in the side of a house; and a house picked up off its foundation and deposited into the middle of the street. I've seen a house cut down the middle from attic to foundation like someone took a giant chainsaw and ripped through it, but nary a picture on the walls was disturbed. I've seen a tornado take out a whole neighborhood of houses and leave one house with only a few broken windows.

Tornado outbreaks are getting worse; not the number of tornadoes, but their intensity and strength, which makes them more dangerous. Whether this has anything to do with global climate change or not is anyone's guess, but my money says it is. I can definitely see the changes in the weather, and of tornadoes in particular, and I've lived with tornadoes my whole life.

The United States leads the world in the number of annual tornadoes, numbering about 1,000. In 2011, the super-outbreak across the Midwest and the South resulted in 362 tornados across the United States; 218 occurred in one day, and 55 of those tornadoes were recorded in the state of Alabama, where they caused about 248 deaths, more than 2,200 injuries, and massive property damage.

Just around breakfast time, my brother Joey heard a sound like a freight train and felt the hairs on his arms stand straight up. He grabbed the kids and put them in the bathtub and covered them with his body. When the tornado had passed, in the bed where six-year-old Michael had been sleeping, a tree now rested. Later in the day, some of Joey's chicken houses were hit, and in the next series of tornadoes, his other chicken houses were hit. He was lucky that all were safe and alive, but it was a hard and stressful time for him and his family, as well as for many families across the country as people worked to recover and rebuild. There are too many stories from that outbreak to tell, some heartbreaking and some miraculous.

During the 2011 outbreak, Scott, an herb student and friend, heard the tornado and ushered his family out of the house to the lowest-lying area, which was a small creek that cut behind the back of their house. All five children were with them, and Scott covered his five-year-old and six-month-old children with his body. His wife Angela did the same with their two- and seven-year-old sons. The eleven-year-old son hunkered between them. When the tornado had passed, their house was fully demolished, and if they had stayed inside, it's a good chance that all would have died. But they were missing one child, the five-year-old daughter who had been ripped from under Scott by the force of the winds. She was later found wrapped in a blanket in a tree, safe and sound, but scared.

The devastation that results from the meeting of the elements that create a tornado doesn't only affect humans and their property. It also affects the natural landscape and the animals that live there. Hundreds and thousands of acres of trees and forests are lost each year to these massive rotating storms. The fibers in the wood of a tree can only bend and give so much before they succumb to the powerful forces of nature.

There is no tree that is tornado-proof. It will suck an oak right out of the ground, root ball and all. A tornado will snap pine trees and lay them on the ground like thrown matchsticks. Of all the trees, the longleaf pine seems to survive the best. These trees bend and sway in the wind, and a young sapling will bend almost to the ground. The frequent thunderstorms and tornados that are common in the Southeast don't affect them like it does their cousins, the loblolly and slash pines. Tornadoes will snap a loblolly into halves and break a slash pine quite easily. But not the longleaf. No sir. This pine bends and sways in the wind, holding onto the ground with all its might with a deep taproot nearly as large in diameter as the trunk. The broad taproot burrows about fifteen feet into the soil, while the lateral roots will radiate between thirty-five and seventy-five feet from the trunk. Grounded to say the least.

There is no rhyme or reason for the randomness of a tornado's selection of destruction or of life. The chaos is the meeting of the natural forces of hot/cold and wet/dry, and it seems that natural law is suspended as the Earth tries to find balance. The result is pressure, irritation, and chaos as the elements try to find equilibrium again, as the Earth tries to find homeostasis. This is true on the land or in the body. When these forces meet in the body, the chaos that prevails is irritation, inflammation, and pain, pretty much the hallmark of chronic disease. That's the meeting of hot/cold and wet/dry.

Hot/cold and wet/dry—these are the properties that can be used to describe the weather, the body, and herbal remedies. Let's explore these concepts in relation to Southern Folk Medicine.

Hot

Hot is associated with blood. Heat denotes the presence of life; cold, its absence. A warm body is a live body: Blood is moving through the vessels, and the chest rises and falls with each breath.

You can observe a feverish child with bright red cheeks and a sweaty brow and know that the blood is involved. It is a fairly simple deduction whether we speak of humoral medicine, Native American medicine, or conventional medicine. Heat can be carried by the air, wind, water, and the rain and dew or food. It can present as hot and damp or hot and dry, both on the land and in the body.

Heat in the body can be caused by too much sun. In a climate where summer temperatures easily reach 100°F for days on end, without the benefit of air conditioning this was a tremendous matter of concern. People could die working out in the fields from sunstroke. Signs of sunstroke include headache, followed by light-headedness and a downward progression from there. Too much sun can touch the mind, cloud the thoughts, and cause stumbling and stuttering. Everyone knew that if you became overheated, you stopped sweating and your body would go into chills. This is dangerous indeed. Nausea, vomiting, and rapid heartbeat followed—at the extreme, death.

Summer's heat can lead to excess sweating and dehydration, which can lead to stroke. Extreme electrolyte imbalance from loss of minerals can lead to heart attack and nervous system disorders.

Heat in the body could also be a sign of infection or illness. A slight fever engages the immune system and kills pathogens. It's the body's natural defense against illness. Children are more prone to fever than adults, and care should be taken to ensure that appropriate fever temperatures are maintained. Caution if the temperature is above 102°F, as children's fevers can spike pretty fast. Bathing a child in lukewarm water can often bring down a fever. In any situation, appropriate fever management should be initiated.

Heat is also symbolic for inflammation. Normally, inflammation, swelling, and white blood cell release are other protective mechanisms of the immune system. When an area becomes inflamed, blood flow increases to that area and may cause redness, a feeling of heat, and pain. Increased swelling is a sign that the body is doing its job to protect the tissues. If you roll your ankle, the increased swelling and inflammation and accompanying pain are present to make sure that you immobilize the injured joint and stop putting weight on it.

Sometimes, heat in the body, the inflammatory process, gets out of control, for example, with fibromyalgia, which causes pain and stiffness in the muscles. Sometimes, inflammation is present because the body is attacking itself, such as in rheumatoid arthritis, lupus, multiple sclerosis, and other autoimmune disorders. Other causes of heat in the body include excess thyroid activity, hives, chronic illnesses, and physical injury or surgery.

Water is an excellent medium to cool down the body's heat. As tissues become dry and blood thickens, water is needed to moisten and cool the body and thin and move the blood. This can include both drinking water and bathing it in. Too much heat in the body creates dryness that affects the kidneys, heart, mucous membrane tissues, and the lungs. In the nervous system, heat is reflected as tremors and twitches, zings, and buzzes.

When the body is hot or when the climate is hot, the appetite is diminished. In the hot summer months, folk's caloric intact is greatly decreased. "It's just too hot to eat," they say. The same is true of fever, inflammation, and other heating of the body. It's best to reduce the intake of food and let the body do its job. As the old saying goes, "Feed a cold and starve a fever." This is good advice whether it's the fever of illness or the elevation of body heat due to the environment.

In hyperthyroidism, the appetite may either increase or decrease as the body searches to balance energy output. In extreme heating conditions such as high fever, the body consumes itself for the nutritional resources required to fight off the infection and lower the fever. This is the primary reason that you can be several pounds lighter after an illness. This is a deficiency state, and the body will require rebuilding.

Matthew Wood, author of *The Practice of Traditional Western Herbalism*, recommends herbal sedatives to reduce the heat of excited tissues, and suggests peach leaf and lemon balm. Personally, I would also add chickweed, passionflower, Solomon's seal, marshmallow, and slippery elm. Extreme heat can cause dryness and atrophy of tissues. Wood suggests nutritive tonics such as milky oats and cleavers.

Interestingly, in European folk medicine, which developed in a cool and damp climate, the danger was making the body too cold because cold meant death. Here in the South, which is a hot and damp climate, it was more important to reduce the heat by any means possible. This is an important point: Folk medicines developed with the geography and climate of the land. While the principles from one folk medicine practice may be applicable to other areas of the world, we must always keep in mind that climate changes from location to location must be taken into account.

The body produces sweat to stay cool. With a hot and humid climate, the increased moisture in the air slows down the evaporative, cooling process. This is known as the heat index. The outside temperature may be 95°F, but the humidity makes it feel like 101°F. When your body can't evaporate the sweat to stay cool, the body temperature rises and heat exhaustion and heat stroke result.

Heat is irritating on the body, mind, and spirit. In cold weather, we can always add another layer of clothing to keep us warm, but in the heat, there are only so many clothes we can take off and still be socially acceptable. Heat zaps our energy and drains us dry. It can cause heart palpitations and electrolyte loss. We can't get enough water, but oddly don't feel like drinking. Tempers are short and the murder rate climbs. In the heat of the moment, people make rash decisions and may have a prickly heat rash on their body. Sex drive drops, activity level drops, and in the middle of the afternoon, folks just sit around and do nothing or nap. Of course, the controlled environment of air conditioning has changed much of this, but not all. I do encourage that if a person works outdoors in the heat, not to have their air conditioning set too low at home. Let the body adjust and give it time to do so by having a little higher indoor temperature, say 76 to 80°F degrees.

Women suffer more in the heat than men, the reverse of winter. Women's bodies are less able to disperse the heat or to cool down as quickly at night due to their subcutaneous layer of fat. Night cooling during the hot summer is important for recuperation, and without it, heat exhaustion and death can occur. Historically, more women have died in heat waves than men, and women are more susceptible to exhaustion, headaches, and fainting in the heat. The summer pulse is not too different from the winter pulse; it is strong and somewhat fast. But in the summer, the pulse is closer to the surface and not as deep.

You'll notice that some of the herbs that were mentioned as heating the body are also included in the cooling section. Herbs that make you sweat can have the effect of cooling the body, depending upon the method of application. For example, in the winter if you take cayenne, it will increase circulation and warm the body, but will not make you sweat due to the relative environmental temperature. A little trick for cold weather is to put cayenne powder in your shoes. It will warm the feet and improve circulation without taking it internally. On the other hand, in the summer when the relative temperature is much, much warmer, taking or eating cayenne will cause you to sweat; the sweat evaporates, creating a cooling effect.

Another little herbal trick: If you drink peppermint, spearmint, or sage tea hot, it warms the body and increases circulation. If you drink the tea at room temperature, it cools the body. So, warm drinks in winter and room temperature drinks in the summer.

Foods may carry heat or cause heat when eaten. Foods that carry heat include any cooked foods or hot beverages. Just a cup of hot water can heat the body and stimulate the digestion and blood. This makes warm drinks good in the winter, but too heating in the summer.

Herbs that reduce fever include blue vervain, black cohosh, skullcap, lobelia, plantain, slippery elm, elder, peppermint, yarrow, boneset, cornsilk, bilberry, and dandelion, to name a few.

Herbs that cool the body, taken as a room-temperature tea, include sumac, sourwood, red raspberry leaves and fruit, ground ivy, peppermint, black cohosh, spearmint, cayenne, blue vervain, catnip, sage, thyme, and all traditional fruits and berries such as peaches, citrus fruits, watermelons, muskmelons, cantaloupe, and other melons.

Cold

Cold is associated with mucus. When it's cold outside, there is a tendency for the body to produce mucus as protection from the irritation. Like heat, cold can be carried by the air, wind, water, and the rain and dew or food. It can be cold and damp or cold and dry; both on the land or in the body. It is associated with an over-relaxed tissue state.

Moving the mucus is of vital importance; mucus that doesn't move causes congestion of an area. Stagnant, constricted, unmoving mucus reduces the flow of blood and lymph, which further perpetuates the stagnation and the ensuing inflammation. Stagnant mucus is the perfect breeding ground for bacteria, whether in the nose, lungs, or gut. Keep that mucus moving!

A cold temperature forces the body to work harder to maintain its core temperature, including shivering to generate heat. Folks will also stamp their feet, flail their arms, and bounce up and down in place to generate heat. Wind chill, a combination of air temperature and wind speed, causes heat to leave the body more rapidly. As the body loses heat, a person may experience confusion, shallow breathing, clumsiness, tiredness, and sleepiness, and ultimately loss of consciousness. The pulse may be weak and irregular, and the heart rate slows. This is an extreme relaxed state. In the early stages, stimulating and heating herbs such as cayenne, cinnamon, cloves, black pepper, ginger, angelica, smartweed, and prickly ash can help keep the blood moving and warm the body.

When the weather is cold, our appetite increases and we tend to eat more. Calories are heat, and when we are cold, whether from the external temperature or internal processes, we'll automatically take in more calories or conserve energy and calories to increase heat. This is why we gravitate toward high-calorie, nutritionally poor food when we are cold or in a nutritionally deficient state; it is quick heat and energy. Eating high-calorie simple carbohydrates to increase heat can also increase an already deficient state. Ideally, we should train ourselves to reach for the nutritionally dense foods such as good protein sources, root vegetables, whole grains, green vegetables, and fruits to help stay healthy and avoid illness. Unfortunately, it's easier to reach for the mashed potatoes, pasta, cakes, pies, and cookies.

Cold can be created in the body as a result of deficiency. The aftereffects and recovery from acute illness, injury, or surgery can drain the body of vital nutrients and vital energy, creating coolness and a deficiency state. As the person begins recovery from the acute condition and regains strength, the blood moves and warmth returns to the limbs and energy to the body.

Cold denotes the absence of life, and this can occur in stages beginning with coolness. Chronic illness, such as hypothyroidism, and other deficiency diseases deplete the body of strength, vitality, and nutrients, leading to cold. The hands are cold, the feet are cold, and the back shivers. Energy is extremely low. The blood isn't moving or is nutritionally poor. The lymph thickens and moves slowly around the body, creating dampness and congestion in vessels and nodes. Blood pressure may be low in the beginning but higher as the heart works to move the blood. The body needs heat, movement, and nutrients for recovery. A warm sweater, a tweak of the thermostat, a walk around the block, or an extra blanket in the evenings are all warranted in this situation. If you are cold, create an artificial warmth until your body can produce its own heat. Continuing to feel cold will only drain you further and create more deficiency.

Cold is sedating on the body, mind, and spirit. The heart and the brain struggle to operate at peak efficiency during cold weather. Cold weather can create isolation as people tend to stay indoors or limit time outdoors. Winter is the traditional time to recharge, reflect, and rest. While humans don't actually hibernate, cold temperatures and shorter days encourage us to stay in and reduce socialization (except for holidays). You may have noticed that during the winter when the days are shorter, you want to sleep longer and require more rest. At 8 p.m. in the winter, you might feel that you are ready for a good night's sleep, while at 8 p.m. in the summer, you are still full of energy. Energy levels are down in winter, the thyroid is busy keeping us warm, and we have little energy to spare for robust activity.

In the winter, men suffer more than women. Men feel the cold less readily than women but can't maintain a constant core temperature quite as easily. Women feel colder sooner but it is a surface cold, a skin cold, and women shiver sooner than men. Women have the ability to maintain a more constant core temperature due to a thicker layer of subcutaneous fat. This difference in how men and women experience cold will be reflected in the pulse. Here, the male pulse may feel strong and somewhat faster as the circulatory system shifts blood flow patterns to accommodate the colder weather by constricting blood vessels. A woman's pulse will feel deeper, but still somewhat fast.

There are more heart attacks in winter. Cold weather makes the heart work harder. It's a good idea, if you work out, to exercise in a heated environment. The heart has to work extra hard to exercise and keep the circulation moving in the winter temperatures. Shoveling snow is not your best form of exercise and is a known trigger for heart attack. Nor is jogging in the freezing cold a good idea either.

Elderly people, who already have sluggish circulation, may feel a slight strain as the heart beats faster to reduce the effects of the cold. Older folks tend to compensate for the cold, on both the brain and the heart, by increasing the temperature in their homes and wearing extra layers of clothes. The blood is a bit thicker due to the cold and age which tends to increase the strain on the heart.

Traditionally, winter was the time of eating stored grains and meats, foods high in fat and salt. Circulating fats in the blood also make for thicker blood. Thick blood slows down blood flow and makes the heart work harder. One of the reasons for the traditional spring cleanse was to thin the blood and move the accumulated winter fats.

Foods can either carry cold or cause cold when eaten. Foods that carry cold include citrus fruits, fruit juices, berries, watermelon, or raw cruciferous vegetables like broccoli and cauliflower. Foods that cause cold when eaten include cream cheese, ice cream, and other dairy products, as well as processed meats, and mayonnaise.

Herbs to offset cold and warm the body are stimulating herbs such as cayenne, lobelia, pine, ginger, cloves, cinnamon, allspice, American ginseng, fennel, fenugreek, black pepper, garlic, horseradish, kelp, prickly ash, anise, sarsaparilla, sassafras, and bay, to name a few.

Wet

Wet, also known as damp, is associated with mucus and other fluids in the body, including lymph, sweat, and urine. Damp is carried by rain, dew, fog, mist, air, wind, and food. Damp itself may carry heat or cold. Cold, damp weather seeps into the body and increases the conduction of heat out of the body. Our clothing soaks up the moisture from the atmosphere and sucks the heat away. It takes more energy to heat water than it does air. So cold, damp air always feels colder than cold, dry air. Blood flow moves deeper into the body to protect the core, and ligaments and tendons tighten. It's a really unpleasant feeling—just the sort to make you long for a nice warm fire and a cup of something hot and steaming.

In the body, infection may cause areas of damp as inflammation increases and fluid moves to critical areas. In some situations, pus may be generated. Parasite infection may cause an irritated damp condition in the small intestines as mucus is generated. Leaky gut, food sensitivities, irritable bowel syndrome, diverticulitis, and ulcerative colitis are all damp conditions and may also carry heat or cold. For example, the inactive diverticulosis is cold and damp and the active diverticulitis is hot and damp.

Lungs, bronchial tubes, and sinus passages are obvious areas of damp. Cold and damp in the lungs may present as pneumonia, emphysema, chronic obstructive pulmonary disease (COPD), or smoker's lungs. Acute pneumonia is hot and damp, while walking pneumonia is cold and damp. Damp conditions can be found in any mucous membrane tissue, including the female reproductive system.

Congestion leads to stagnation due to constricted blood and lymph flow. Damp leads to an over-relaxed state. Think about the gallbladder for a moment, which is a muscular sack lined with mucous membrane tissue. The gallbladder receives bile from the liver and then releases it into the small intestine during the digestive process. Bile is irritating on mucous membrane tissues and creates mucus in the gallbladder. The gallbladder fills and fills with mucus and bile (sludge), and loses the ability to contract. This is a damp, over-relaxed state. Herbs to initiate contraction of the gallbladder, such as yellow dock, wild yam, dandelion, goldenseal, Solomon's seal, yellow root, fenugreek, fennel, and yucca can move the damp and tone the tissues.

Kidney, liver, and cardiovascular disorders can also cause dampness and the accumulation of fluid in various parts of the body. If there is kidney dysfunction or disease, fluid may accumulate in feet, ankles and hands, which is generally cold and damp. As the kidney disease worsens, there may be shortness of breath, fatigue, and decreased urination and accumulation of fluid in the abdomen (cold and damp). The accumulation of fluid in the abdomen is known as ascites and may also be present in liver disease and congestive heart failure (cold and damp).

Cold and damp are much more common in the body than hot and damp. Damp (water) tends to have a cooling effect in general. However, fever and high inflammation tend to turn cold and damp into hot and damp.

Damp may also be present in the lymphatic system as the result of lack of movement or disease. For example, think about the accumulation of fluid in your midsection and upper thighs from sitting all day or flying on an airplane. Illnesses that limit lymph flow such as mononucleosis also create damp. Hypothyroidism, chronic viral infections, allergies, ovarian cysts, and enlarged prostate are other examples of the presence of damp.

Chronic stress is one of the most common reasons I see for damp. In this situation, digestion shuts down. The survival reasoning is simple: The body can't be eating and digesting and running and fighting all at the same time. Because digestive activity is diminished, foods pass more slowly through the digestive tract, creating damp and bloating. When a person is under chronic stress and taking antibiotics, this is a double-damp whammy on the digestive tract.

Foods may carry damp or cause damp when eaten. For example, ice cream, oatmeal, soups, mashed potatoes, and refried beans carry damp. Any dairy product causes damp, including yogurt, kefir, and other fermented dairy. Raw nuts and seeds and dried fruits can cause damp.

Herbs that tone the tissues or have astringent activity, diuretics, and stimulants can help move damp: red raspberry, sumac, mullein, marshmallow, black walnut, white oak bark, hydrangea, chickweed, Queen Anne's lace, sage, Queen of the Meadow, ginger, yellow dock, red root, and lobelia, to name a few.

Dry

Dry is the lack of fluid. In dry conditions, there is little or no moisture. "Dry as a bone" is an old saying to describe a total lack of available moisture. It can be cold and dry or hot and dry, both on the land or in the body. Dry is carried by the air, wind, and food.

Cold, dry air in the winter pulls moisture from the body and chaps the skin and lips. Hot, dry air pulls moisture from the body and dries the skin, lips, and hair. If the humidity is extremely low, the sweat will evaporate as soon as the body releases it. In this climate, it's prudent to drink vast amounts of water because it is very easy to become dehydrated even though you aren't aware of the sweat. Wearing a hat in a hot, dry climate will shield and protect your head and eyes from the effects of a boiling sun, but may or may not keep your head cooler, even though it may feel cooler.

Fever may create hot and dry tissues in the body. Here, as with external heat, staying hydrated is extremely important. The cooling herbs mentioned above can help lower fever and conserve internal moisture. A bit of fruit juice mixed in water may improve ingestion of the water and improve hydration.

Wasting diseases, such as extreme hyperthyroidism, end-stage cancer, HIV infections, tuberculosis, autoimmune diseases, and chronic infections, can cause hot and dry conditions in the body and ultimately tissue atrophy. In this situation, the body is consuming itself at an alarming rate, regardless of the number of calories consumed. Often at this stage, the person is continually craving processed sugar and simple carbohydrates as the disease demands more and more glucose for cell division, hence the old saying, "Sugar feeds cancer." In some disease conditions, not only is the body wasting from lack of nutrition in the disease, but fever is simultaneously ravaging the body.

Dry is mediated by water and other fluid intake, since dry is often associated with lack of moisture. However, dry can also result from lack of oil. Our bodies rely on adequate fat intake, especially omegas-3 and -6, for the creation of a strong cell membrane, reproductive hormones, skin and hair health, and fat-soluble vitamins. Healthy oils also help reduce inflammation, improve brain health, and reduce risk for cardiovascular disease.

Foods that are dry include popcorn without butter, cornbread, breads, rice, most any grains, dried fruits and vegetables, and potatoes. Folks with a dry esophagus should be especially cautious, as dry foods can trigger esophageal spasms or contractions. We commonly add oil, butter, or dairy to moisten dry foods.

Herbs to improve dry include moistening and oily herbs, such as Solomon's seal, fennel, fenugreek, yucca, mullein, marshmallow, kelp, red clover, hydrangea, alfalfa, hens and chickens, chickweed, okra, and angelica.

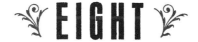

EIGHT

The Constitutions

I ate no butcher's meat, lived chiefly on fruits, vegetables, and fish, and never drank a glass of spirits or wine until my wedding day. To this I attribute my continual good health, endurance, and an iron constitution.

—John James Audubon

AS MENTIONED EARLIER, folk medicines developed with the geography and climate of the land. While the principles from one folk medicine practice may be applicable to other areas of the world, we must always keep in mind that climate changes from location to location must be taken into account. One climate may be hot and dry, while another is hot and damp, cold and damp, or cold and dry.

It doesn't matter where on this Earth you live, the geography of the land shapes your health. For me and mine, it has been the geography of the American Southeast, hot and humid, the perfect environment for thousands of species of plants to make their homes. My ancestors must have found this land a veritable natural supermarket abounding with herbs, fruits, vegetables, and wild game.

In North America, the climate is as changeable as the air; hot and cold and wet and dry come together on this spot of Earth in unique weather patterns such as tornadoes, raging storms, hurricanes, and brutal heat. Here it is altogether a different climate than the even, cool dampness of the British Isles and Northern Europe where air, water, and earth meet in a more stable and genteel fashion.

The settlers changed the landscape of the New World as forests were cut and land was cleared in the attempt to re-create what had been left behind in Europe. The Celts had little reason to work this hard and blended into the mountains and hills with their rough cabins and slight gardens in a more natural fashion. Their crop was hard liquor, which required little changing of the land but a swift foot to avoid the revenuers, agents of the U.S. Treasury Department.

On the surface, the land was transformed into farms and settlements, and later into towns and cities. However, a constant tug with Mother Nature and the climate is still felt as she continually tries to reclaim what once was, to return the landscape to the geography best suited to the elements. Rain must flow and drain or it becomes a flood. Wind must flow around pressure systems so that we can feel the Earth turn beneath us. And lightning must flash whether around buildings or dense forests. We humans have changed the course of rivers, leveled mountains, irrigated deserts, and mined deep into the ground, all in an attempt to master and control our mutual home, Mother Earth.

The land of my ancestors shapes my health as surely as any other influence. Regardless of where you now live, the original land of your ancestors is intricately bound in your DNA, molding who you are, how healthy you are, what foods are the most nutritionally sound for you, and ultimately what you will pass to your children. Most of this is contained in our DNA and epigenetic code, and some is in our mitochondrial DNA. A good question to ask is, "Where do my people come from?"

It is the health of the land that shapes us, both the land upon which we now live and the land of our ancestors. It affects and gives shape to our constitutions. Your nuclear DNA, shaped as a double helix, is the repository of your genetic material passed by your ancestors to your parent and then to you—twenty-three genes received from your mother and twenty-three genes from your father. Your genes are fixed, and their required stability and ability to repair when damaged are absolutely necessary for the continuation of your genetic line. Have you ever been looking through the family photos and noticed that your brother looks like your great-great uncle? Or that you have your great-grandmother's nose? Or that your child has her great-great-great grandfather's forehead? It's always a roll of the genetic dice.

Stability of genetic material forms the basis of your constitution. A variation in your genetic code creates your individual susceptibility or risk to various diseases across your lifespan, including issues such as type 2 diabetes, autoimmune disorders, Parkinson's disease, and cancers. But your genes may also pass genetic diseases, such as cystic fibrosis and sickle cell anemia.

And then, there's the mitochondrial DNA (mtDNA), shaped in a circle, that we inherit only from our mothers. It is less stable and not as fixed or complex as our nuclear DNA, but also contributes to our constitutional makeup. Mitochondria serve the function of creating energy within the cells; we can't live without them. Your ability to convert food into energy is directly due to your inheritance of mtDNA from your mother. How we make cellular energy and the amount we make are directly linked to our supply of Vital Energy, our ch'i. If our mothers have strong Vital Energy, then there's a good bet that we will too.

Because we inherit our mtDNA from our mothers, it is not unique for each individual, since all the maternal relatives have identical mtDNA sequences. In other words, you have the same mtDNA as your mother, grandmother, great-grandmother, and all the other grandmothers all the way back to the original female in your line. Through mtDNA, scientists can trace your lineage back to your ancient, ancient ancestors. An mtDNA lineage ends when a mother has no daughters.

(I find it very interesting and equally amazing that historically many Native American tribes had a matriarchal culture. Women owned the house and land and had control over the children. Inheritance was through the female line, not the male lineage. This makes perfect sense when we think about the circular mtDNA because it is only passed through the female line.)

After death, nuclear DNA degrades very rapidly and little can be found in decomposed remains. But not so the mtDNA! It can be found in high numbers within the cells and is more likely than nuclear DNA to survive after a long period of time because its circular shape makes it less vulnerable to degradation and adds to its stability. Scientists can use mtDNA of various populations to map out the ancestry and migration routes of ancient humans. Very interesting.

But that's not the last influence of genetics in our constitutional makeup. Now we come to the role of epigenetics. It seems that we have a third biological code that affects our health, happiness, and behavior. Nuclear DNA sets our individual, fixed genetics. No two people are exactly alike unless you are identical twins. Mitochondrial DNA forms the framework of our energy and health. And epigenetics reveals the dynamic, fluid potential of our nuclear DNA and mtDNA.

The epigenetic code is determined by the methylation of DNA, which can turn genes on or off and controls when and where information is given to the cells. Epigenetics can be influenced by physical and emotional trauma, environmental toxins, nutritional status, and stress, especially in childhood. These influences create tags of information that are attached to the outside of the DNA and are then inherited by a person's offspring. It can have an impact across several generations.

Epigenetic tags may increase risk of cancers, cause birth defects, and affect a person's mental health. They can affect obesity, risk for cardiovascular disease and type 2 diabetes, and other disorders. Epigenetic tags are influenced first and foremost by nutrition. Certain nutrients, particularly vitamins B6, folate, B12, selenium, zinc, calcium, and magnesium, along with sulfur-containing amino acids, can reverse or change epigenetic tags and improve DNA methylation. This has the effect of modifying the expression of genes that affect many processes, including embryonic development, aging, and cancer risk. Epigenetic changes can be inherited during cell division, passing the change down through the generations. But remember: Epigenetics doesn't change your nuclear DNA; it only creates a new tag of information that wraps around the outside of the DNA, which are then inherited.

How many generations of epigenetic tags are inherited? That's a really interesting question that doesn't have an answer at this point. Studies have shown three or four generations is common. But at what point can epigenetic changes become permanent? That is another good question without a solid answer. I prefer to think about the concept of the Native American Seven Generations: Make your decisions based on behalf of the seven generations still to come. That seems about right to me.

As you can see, our constitutional makeup begins in the womb, includes our nuclear DNA, our mitochondrial DNA, and any epigenetic tags that are inherited. But it is more than what we are born with. Constitutional influences include early childhood influences, with diet and nurturing especially crucial. Or put another way, our nature plus our nurture.

Our constitutional makeup includes our physical strengths and weaknesses, emotional balance, mental health stability, and spiritual awareness. It acknowledges our family health history, both physical and psychological, our personal life history, lifestyle factors that affect health, childhood upbringing and illnesses, and social and cultural factors that influence our health and mental well-being.

In addition, our constitution includes conditions our mother experienced during pregnancy, including her diet, lifestyle factors, exposure to environmental toxins, any use of medications or recreational drugs, her stress level and emotional health, physical activity and exercise level, and sleeping patterns. During pregnancy, our mother's blood is our blood. The food she eats creates our bodies. The nutrients she intakes are the basic building blocks of us. This is a huge responsibility, and one that should not be taken lightly.

Our constitutional makeup continues to develop until about the age of six or seven. Some people have iron-clad constitutions and never seem to be sick a day in their lives. They are filled with energy, never miss a day of work, and somehow have the energy to run marathons on the weekends and bake cookies for their child's class. Other folks have delicate or sensitive constitutions and have trouble navigating a shopping trip due to the onslaught of odors and fragrances. Their low energy levels require great attention to their lifestyle choices and social activities.

A person's constitutional makeup isn't an indicator of longevity or happiness, but offers guidelines to staying well and may indicate health challenges or tendencies a person might face throughout their lifespan. Knowing your possible health challenges creates a wonderful opportunity for heading them off at the pass. Once you are aware of your constitutional makeup, the trick is then to follow the guidelines that can help keep your constitution in balance or bring it back to balance in times of stress or illness.

This awareness can help you create and follow a personal health plan. Also, actively pursuing knowledge of your constitutional makeup opens health education opportunities as you investigate dietary suggestions and potential allergens, try out different exercise options, and find your best stress relief modality.

The bottom line: Understanding your constitutional makeup helps you make the most of what you've got.

Southern Folk Constitutions and Elements

As a folk medicine based on oral tradition, the language and vocabulary of Southern Folk Medicine are metaphorical ones, based on the common language of the people. As discussed earlier in the text, blood is considered the most important fluid in the body. The characteristics observed in the blood describe the state of physical health. The state of mucus is also important, as is that of the nerves, but neither is as easily observable as blood. We get cut and we bleed. This is immediately observable. Is it thick or thin? Dry or wet? Red or purple? Mucus is less easy to observe unless we think of mucus production during a cold or excreting mucus through our colon due to an irritation. But what about all the internal mucus, fluids, and extracellular matrix that we can't see? And the state of the nerves is only observable through our actions, movements, personality, and thoughts.

In Southern Folk Medicine, there are four elements: fire, water, air, and earth. These are basic environmental factors. Ask any forest ranger. Life on this planet will quickly die without air or water. There is no life without the home the Earth provides. And fire in the forest, even through natural means such as lightning strikes, well, that's a different story, but a necessary one.

Fire converts one form of energy in the forest into another, as so within our bodies. When a tree burns, the organic and inorganic compounds within it are transformed and percolate into the soil to be used by other trees or plants. Fire in the forest is an ancient factor bound up in the evolution of plants. Some trees, such as those with serotinous cones like the lodgepole pine or sequoia, germinate only after fire has cracked open the seed cone.

A healthy forest is a balanced combination of these four elements, as is the human body. When these four elements are harmonious, there is abundant life. When they are balanced in the body, there is good health. In Southern Folk Medicine, the four elements are written as pairs of opposites: fire/water and air/earth. There are four tastes, bitter, salty, sour, and sweet, also written in pairs of opposites: bitter/salty and sour/sweet.

The four elements and four tastes are used, metaphorically, to describe the four main constitutions in Southern Folk Medicine—Bitter Blood, Salty Blood, Sour Blood, and Sweet Blood. These are also written in pairs of opposites: Bitter/Salty Blood and Sour/Sweet Blood.

Each element—fire, earth, air, and water—corresponds to a Southern Blood Type and helps describe its physical and psychological traits. Bitter Blood is fire. Salty Blood is water. Sour Blood is air. And Sweet Blood is earth. Please understand that the term *element* is not used in this context in relation to chemistry. Here, it is used to describe components of composition or influencing factors. It just happens that these components are based on an ancient system that existed before the periodic table.

All four elements operate with us every day. Metaphorically speaking, fire creates energy from the digestion of nutrients; we are about 70 percent water; we breathe air; and our bones are made of minerals from the Earth.

We are all born with all elements within us. We are a composite in every sense of the word. Sometimes, an element may dominate in the personality over the others, and this will be readily apparent in our thoughts, actions, habits, and possibly our build. A person might be a Bitter Blood type, which means the element of fire dominates. But that person might also have air, water, and earth, in descending order. Therefore, we must look at the combination of elements in order to understand the whole person; not a single element.

Some folks might have two Southern Blood Types that share equal influence in the personality. For example, a person might have Salty Blood (water) and Sour Blood (air) in equal influence, and then Bitter and Sweet Blood. When two elements dominate in equal amounts, it will manifest in the personality equally also.

Sometimes, a person might have three Southern Blood Types in their constitutional makeup but be missing a fourth. That doesn't mean that the element has no influence in your life; every one of us has all four elements within us. It does mean that the missing element is not apparent in the personality. There are many permutations or combinations that can occur. Again, keep in mind that it is the makeup, the combination, that is important, not just the dominance of one over the other.

No element exists alone. In some way, each one depends upon the other for existence. Fire requires air and earth (fuel) to exist. Water needs earth as a vessel, and air can move water (think rain or storms). Air needs water and earth for existence. And earth, well, houses it all and doesn't need anything to exist. We'll discuss this in more detail in the chapters on each individual element and blood type.

Regardless of whether you have a dominant element or not, you are composed of all four elements and each influences you in some way. Fire governs various processes, especially those related to energy production, hormones, and creativity and passion. Water is concerned with composition of fluids and the removal of wastes; on the emotional level, water is concerned with relationships and feelings. Air is concerned with the brain, the nervous system, and our intellect and ideas. Earth is concerned with the structure of our bones, organ systems, and how we view security and safety.

Going to the Opposite

The descriptions of the blood are based on a system of opposites. For example, blood may be high/low, good/bad, clean/dirty, slow/fast, thick/thin, sweet/sour, or bitter/salty. Keep in mind that these pairs of opposites are just that, opposite ends of a spectrum. If we imagine a line graph with 0 on one end and 10 on the other, the needle, at any given moment, could be anywhere between those numbers depending upon our health and what is happening in our lives. Somewhere, right about center or 5 on our imaginary graph, is the balance, or being just right.

When the elements are in balance, a person exhibits good health. Problems arise when an element becomes out of balance, in either deficiency or excess. When a dominant element or blood type is out of balance in deficiency, the person may exhibit traits of the opposite element. This is an important concept in Southern Folk Medicine—when under stress, we go to our opposite. For example, deficient water may look like fire to some degree. If you don't have enough water, everything is hotter and drier. This is true whether we are talking about the land or the body. When water is deficient, tissues lose their fluidity, and so does the personality. From this point of view, the signs of deficient water element can also be viewed to some extent as characteristics of fire, and vice versa. This will also be true of the pair air/earth.

Stress, illness, or trauma can stretch and strain a person and send them to their opposite element or blood type. Let's look at a person who is predominately Bitter Blood or fire, who is faced with a tight deadline on a project at work. The person begins working long hours, often not taking the time to eat, sitting for long periods, and becoming very critical of those around them. Anger and irritability seem to be the continual presentation in the personality. Automatically, increased fire characteristics will aid the effort to finish the project by the deadline. The person exhibits increased energy at work as the fire rises, but at home, this shift takes a toll with poor-quality sleep and changes in appetite, often with weight gain. The increased energy comes with a price: depletion of nutrients, inability to calm and sleep, and a controlling manner.

As the deadline approaches and success doesn't seem certain, exhaustion and pressure take their toll, and the fire person will begin to express characteristics of its opposite—water. Emotional attachment to the project, tears, and the feeling of being the victim arise. When this happens, the fire or Bitter Blood type is now exhausted, totally stressed, and deficient in vital nutrients. In this example, going to the opposite element of water is viewed as a deficiency state of the fire persona.

A person can stay in a deficiency state for long periods of time. The energy required to hold that position, to hold the opposite element or nature, creates even more deficiency. A person can wallow in their opposite for years, and this can become quite a rut, creating physical, mental, and emotional damage. Being in your opposite will take a huge toll, physically and emotionally, as the body and mind struggle to maintain some sort of equilibrium. We'll discuss herbs and foods to help bring balance in the individual chapters on Southern Blood Types and elements.

When a person goes to their opposite, such as fire to water, it's not a full-blown manifestation of the other element. The fire person will never be as watery as a water person. An air person going to their opposite of earth will never be as grounded and earthy as an earth person. It's all a matter of degree, but it is definitely a noticeable shift.

As you can see, it's always handy to review the opposite element when investigating ongoing patterns of dysfunction or personality changes. Just as we each carry both light and dark within, so do we carry our opposite element.

Comparison to Astrology

I'm often asked if the constitution is the same as the astrological sun sign. The answer is sometimes yes and sometimes no. However, if folks will look deeper into their astrological charts and take into account not only their sun sign, but also moon and ascendant, then I've seen a greater correlation. Back to those signs in the heavens.

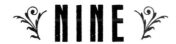

NINE

Fire: Bitter Blood

The spread of civilisation may be likened to a fire; first,
a feeble spark, next a flickering flame, then a mighty blaze,
ever increasing in speed and power.

—*Nikola Tesla*

A MEMORY THAT stands out from my early childhood days is the day Daddy got fired from his job. We rented a rundown house from Mr. Scofield that was set back in the woods. It was down a dirt road, not even a graveled one. Not only was the road total dirt, so was the front yard—the sandy soil with little pebbles that is common in parts of north Alabama. Mama was outside sweeping the yard when Daddy came home from work. This was a daily task and I had my own little broom to help.

In those days, it was common practice to keep the front yard totally devoid of grass, only bare dirt. Each day Mama swept that dirt yard as clean as if it were the living room. The marks left by the broom in the sandy soil had a mesmerizing pattern that I found comforting. I could sit and watch her sweep and never move a muscle; it was almost hypnotic. I've since discovered that many cultures share the tradition of sweeping the yard, such as those from Japan, Africa, Thailand, Mexico, and Italy. Most likely, this Southern tradition came from Africa.

The stroke used for sweeping the yard is totally different from the stroke used to sweep floors. In the yard, a long, regular stroke was preferred as the goal of sweeping was to remove small debris and leaf bits and leave a fine and smooth broom pattern in its place. Some people used dogwood, some broom sedge, and others used pine. We most often used pine or broom sedge, and sometimes Mama would start with pine and end with sedge, which left a really fine pattern.

Sweeping the yard is not hard work, and doesn't require a lot of muscle. It does require patience and an attentive, meditative state of mind. Your eye must be constantly on the pattern with total absorption and inner concentration for the result of the sweep to be useful. As a child, sweeping the yard taught me a patience that wasn't inherent in my nature or constitution. I had to slow down and just be with the sweeping, and that bit of training has helped me over the years. When I finished helping Mama sweep, there was neatness and order left behind and the world felt right.

Although the yard was dirt all the way around the house, the front yard contained the largest portion of ungrassed yard. Regardless, it all had to be swept. And then there were the flowers. Mama loved her flower beds and each one was neat and weed-free and full of plants, most of which had been given to her by another woman in the community or saved from seed the year before. She was always giving away flower plants and having plants given to her. Her flower beds might contain twenty or thirty different kinds of flowering plants unlike today's mono-plant landscaping style. And then there were all the potted plants that were here and there on both porches. A pot for a plant was anything that might hold dirt and water, from a store-bought pot to an old, painted oil can.

Sweeping the yard allowed you to see the tracks of any person or animal that treaded upon your land. Mama liked sweeping the front yard before sun-down so that, first thing in the morning, we could see what traveled across our yard during the night. We were especially looking for snake tracks. Snakes have a habit of following mice into the house and one time, Mama found a snake (non-poisonous) under her dresser all coiled and stinky. For those that don't know, when snakes are scared, they emit strong odors. The odors can range from musky and strong, which is the odor I most identify with snakes, to sweet or rotting. A few times, I've actually smelled the snake before I saw it.

I would like to say that snakes coming in the house aren't as much of an issue since building styles have changed to closed foundations. But that wouldn't be true. At least with an open foundation, snakes had nowhere hidden to lair or cool off during the summer, and now they do. Just last week one of my daughter's friends opened their oven door to find a snake. A construction friend of mine was remodeling a house last winter and found a rattlesnake hibernating in the wall below the electric box.

Snakes tend to follow the food supply, and if you have mice in the house, then there's a good chance a snake will follow, or at least try, if not into the house, at least to lie in wait somewhere close outside the house. They will also follow chipmunks as a food source. When I was about five, I had two little baby chickens that I kept in a chicken wire cage on the back porch on top an old table. One morning I went out to feed the chicks and a snake had crawled into the cage during the night and eaten them, but was stuck in the wire and couldn't get back out. Daddy made short work of the snake, but my little peeps were gone. I cried and cried, but that is the reality of living close to nature. Everything eats something.

Chickens are good snake control, and when a chicken finds a snake, the alarm is given and the whole flock responds. Guinea hens and turkeys are especially aggressive against snakes, and both will eat small snakes with a gobble. When a chicken finds a snake, it's a tag-team event; usually one chicken, often the rooster, will keep the snake's attention at the front while the flock is pecking away at the back. It's a little scary to see the frenzy of a flock of hens on a snake. Makes me glad they are so small.

Guinea hens going after a snake is a wild, noisy, steroid-driven event. Just stay out of their way. If the chickens can't kill a snake, they will chase it away. Add the barking dogs into the process and it makes for quite a show. When the foundations of houses were on rocks and not enclosed, both the dogs and the chickens wouldn't hesitate to follow the snakes under the house and take care of business.

After the front yard was swept, only the back door was used if we needed to go outside for any reason. The driveway came to the back door, not the front, so any visitors entered the house through the kitchen. Often as not, the visitor just stopped at the kitchen table for a cup of coffee and a visit.

Whatever animal that moved across the dirt yard left a print that was very plain to see. My grandfather once showed me the tracks of a snake which had slithered across the yard sometime between one sweeping and the next. Snake tracks were the most important to look for, the most urgent to find. Nobody wanted snakes in their house. Daddy and Uncle Hastel showed me raccoon tracks, coyote tracks, skunk tracks, and deer tracks. Hastel was a good tracker and knew the tracks very well. The dirt yard was not a place that animals dwelled or hung about for any reason, so it was more like a dirt road for wildlife. Since there wasn't any grass for forage or hiding, there was no reason to linger.

One morning there were human footprints across the yard, which caused my mother a bit of anxiety. It was so hot and no one had air conditioning in those days except the very rich. We slept with our doors and windows wide open to catch any available breeze. Only my parents had a small fan on their dresser to move the air. Us kids just sweated the night away. The screen door was latched, but that wasn't a determent for anyone. Odd that no one was afraid; times have really changed. We didn't have anything to steal except food, but it did happen a couple of times that someone entered the house while we were gone and cooked themselves a cake of cornbread and some eggs and left the dirty dishes. Mama was not pleased.

Because insects need the grass and tall weeds to thrive and the bit of moisture they hold, the open dirt yard created somewhat of an insect barrier leading up to the front porch. Well, except for gnat season, because gnats like to reproduce in sandy soil. The sandy soil covered red clay, and when it rained, the front yard became a muddy mess that was totally avoided by anyone with any common sense. There were a few stepping stones placed in a haphazard fashion from the front porch to the mail box, but it didn't take long for them to be covered in mud too.

Standing out in the freshly swept front yard, it seemed like the whole world changed with the words that Daddy said: "I've been fired." To my young mind, this sounded horrendous. Did someone hold Daddy down and blast a blowtorch in his face? Did his boss set the seat of Daddy's overalls on fire? These were the images that moved through my mind. Being fired seemed like a frightening and violent thing to happen. I was to come to know that this wouldn't be the last time we heard those words from Daddy, "I've been fired," or the other, which was almost as bad, "I've been laid off."

Up until this point in my life, fire had a totally different connotation and was strictly a noun, unless you applied the word "fire" to the discharge of a gun. You built a fire in the fireplace or cast-iron stove. You burned the leaves in the yard. You burned the woods to get rid of the underbrush and ticks. Lightning struck a house and burned it down. A chimney caught on fire and burned down the house. When you'd done something really bad, Mama would take a hickory switch and set your britches on fire. A randy person was hot to trot. A roll of good luck was a hot streak. A female dog went into heat. A tie game was a dead heat. A person who acted impulsive acted in the heat of the moment.

Daddy would say, "Get under this shade tree out of the heat." And one of my Aunt Sadie's favorites, "If you can't take the heat, get out of the kitchen," and she meant this both figuratively and literally. In the summertime, we often had a heat wave. And sometimes, we had to fight fire with fire. Mama would yell at my sister "to light a fire under those feet and get moving." And where's there's smoke, there has to be fire. And so on. It makes for a colorful language.

Fire was necessary to our existence and such a common element in our language that numerous idioms abound for almost any instance that heat or fire best illustrate the situation. But this was the first time I had heard "fired" used as a verb in this manner. I just didn't know what it meant.

As soon as Daddy said those words, "I've been fired," Mama stood stock still, then slumped a little and very pitifully and sadly, and with long emphasis and pain said, "Oh, Honey?" It was both a cry and a question. Honey is what Mama called Daddy. She only used his name, Stancel, when she was upset, we were at church or out somewhere, or talking to visitors. At home, he was Honey. The pitiful sound of her voice made me want to go beat up the mean man who had set fire to my Daddy.

I found out later that getting fired meant that Daddy had lost his job. He was around the house a bit more but spent time out looking for work and took on whatever odd job he could find. To make some money, Daddy spent more time in the woods hunting herbs with the family, and often I was able to go with him. Even after he found another construction job, Daddy kept on herb hunting because we were so behind on the bills. Mama worked the Scofield's cotton fields to make some money and took in ironing. It wasn't our last tough time.

Mama never understood or appreciated the value of herbs, but Daddy's family did. They'd always been herb hunters, especially of pink root and American ginseng, but any wild herb they could sell on the market to a company.

A typical ginseng hunt might include Daddy, Granddaddy Light, Uncle Waylon, Aunt Jewel, and Aunt Julie and Uncle Willie. However, Aunt Julie and Uncle Willie preferred sitting along the creek bank fishing while everyone else scampered around the mountain sides. We'd park at the creek and walk up the mountain and hunt along the way. If they'd had luck catching, we'd have fish for supper. It was a fun time.

Aunt Jewel was notorious for wearing metal stove pipes on her legs, in a similar fashion to shin guards, and Army boots on her feet to avoid getting bitten by a snake. She did make a bit of a comical character; she was tall and thin, with gray bobbed hair, and wore an old dress with pants under it, Army boots, and stove pipes. Aunt Jewel would often say that she could hear a snake strike against the pipes but she just kept on walking. Regardless, she was pretty brazen in the woods and would charge through low growth like nobody's business.

Two herbs in Southern Folk Medicine heat the body efficiently but in different ways. American ginseng builds slow heat in the body by working deep within the endocrine system to build energy and endurance. With an appropriate dose, American ginseng is both gentle and effective, and doesn't create jitters or affect sleeping. The building of slow heat brings renewed vigor and vitality, improves endurance, improves sleeping quality, increases the sex drive, and improves memory. The bitter qualities and taste of American ginseng will cause a release of bile that can help improve digestion and facilitate a bowel movement. According to tradition, there isn't a system in the body that ginseng doesn't affect. It is the chief of all herbs.

A dose of American ginseng that is too high in a deficient person will actually force glands and processes into activity that creates more deficiency. A long-lasting fire is built slowly, starting with kindling, and as the fire becomes stronger, more fuel is added. If you use too much wood all at once or logs that are too big, you will smother the fire instead of supporting it. The same with American ginseng—start slow and gently build for a sustained fire.

On the other hand, cayenne creates a blaze of heat by quickly stimulating the movement of blood, opening capillaries, equalizing blood pressure, and sending blood toward the skin's surface. It's almost impossible to take enough ginseng to sweat, but quite easy to take enough cayenne to sweat up a storm—cayenne heats the body. It stimulates the liver, aids digestion, helps heal the digestive tract, and can help lower high cholesterol. Cayenne reduces pain both taken internally and applied topically as a liniment or salve. It stops bleeding, both internally and externally.

Cayenne improves poor circulation, especially in the elderly. In the winter, cayenne taken internally can help warm cold feet and hands by improving blood flow into the extremities of the body, such as the hands, feet and head. Applied topically to swollen, painful joints, cayenne brings blood to the area, reducing pain and turning the skin red. Cayenne, after all, is all about blood.

Using cayenne is like throwing gasoline on the fire. If there's even an ember present, cayenne will stoke it up.

The old saying is, "Cayenne at the start of a heart attack to thin the blood and reduce damage. Ginseng afterward to recover from the heart attack and every day after to stave off another one."

The Heat of the Matter

First and foremost: Fire is hot; heat is the nature of this element. It can be hot and damp or hot and dry, but fire always produces heat.

What is fire? Using the most basic definition, the noun *fire* is the rapid loss of oxygen of a flammable material during the process of combustion. The combustion happens so quickly that it gives off heat, light, and flame. The two basic ingredients needed for a fire are a material that will ignite and oxygen. Fire will only be contained or continue as long as these two elements are present. In other words, fire is an oxidative process.

The element of fire is central to our civilization. Origin stories about fire in indigenous populations and in the mythology of ancient civilizations either view fire as a gift from the gods or something stolen from the gods. Regardless, fire was considered mystical, magical, and spiritual. In some Native American mythology, either crow, water spider, or opossum stole or brought fire from the thunder beings who lived in the sky. In Greek mythology, the Titan Prometheus gave humans the gift of fire. Later the Romans used the deadly Greek fire or war fire to subdue enemies. Its exact composition has remained a secret, but its devastating effects are well recorded in history.

Regardless of its origins, fire changed humanity. With fire, humans were able to cook their meat, which improved digestion and increased available energy. Before fire, all food, including meat, had to be eaten raw. Raw meat and starchy tubers needed to be pounded, or possibly naturally fermented, to be digestible. Cooking allowed our ancestors to gain more energy from their food, which led to increased brain size and other physical adaptations.

Fire provided light, which allowed our ancestors to stay up later at night and continue the activities required for living. It provided warmth in cold weather. Fire also provided a central point for socialization, and that really hasn't changed that much today. Boy Scouts, church groups, campers, indigenous peoples, and social folks of any ilk understand the attraction of sitting around a campfire, sharing stories, singing, and relaxing. There is also something about a fireplace that is comforting and soothing. A fire draws folks together, whether due to its warmth, light, or cheerfulness. There is something about flames that immediately draws the eyes.

Fire often misbehaves. A ground fire can spread faster and burn hotter when moving uphill. There are several reasons for this. When going up the hill, the flames are closer to the fuel (grass, wood, leaves, brush) and dry the fuel out in advance of the flame which makes it ignite more quickly. In addition, as the air heats, the wind currents push up the hill, adding flame to the fire and causing a draft. This draft increases the rate of spread of burning embers, which can then roll downhill starting new fires. And so it spreads. The reverse is also true: A fire spreads slower and burns cooler moving down a hill.

Folks with primary fire constitutions are often the same, burning brighter when the finish line is in sight, running faster up the hill than down it, and blazing at the finish. This is true whether the finish line is related to the completion of a project or an athletic event. Fire people know how to push, and this works as long as they are taking care of themselves and don't have too many irons in the fire.

In the forest, fires help maintain a natural balance among various plant species, certain trees, and the insects and animals dependent upon them for food and shelter. A forest, after all, is a complete ecosystem, not just a bunch of trees stuck together. A natural forest fire only happens when certain conditions are right, when forest moisture and leaf and needle litter are at a certain quantity and quality level. Because conditions have to be just right, the frequency and intensity of a natural forest fire is mandated by the forest itself. If artificially created outside of the ecosystem's natural timing, forest fires can burn hotter and more intense, causing more harm than benefit.

The same is also true of fire people. As long as their fire, or energy production, is flowing along natural time cycles related to a healthy endocrine system, the fire person is happy, productive, and accomplishes much. If they try to artificially stoke their fire by eating too many carbohydrates or taking recreational drugs, then a health disaster awaits as their innate fire sputters and crashes.

The temperature of a fire depends upon the type of fuel in the fire, how much oxygen is available, and the moisture content of the burning material. The cooler the flame (red, blue), the more incomplete the combustion and the more soot and particles that are produced. The hotter the flame (white, yellow), the more complete the combustion and less ash or soot that is produced. A hotter flame is a cleaner burn, producing fewer free radicals and indicating complete combustion. This is also true in energy production within the cells.

This is an important point for fire folk. The amount of energy produced from food is going to depend on the type and quantity of food in the diet. While this is a true statement for everyone, regardless of constitution, it is extremely important for the fire constitution. Too much food, especially simple carbohydrates, and the system is overwhelmed. Too little food and there isn't enough food for fueling. Finding the quantity and type of food that creates energy is extremely important.

In general, fire people do well with good-quality fats and proteins, vegetables, beans, and fruits and nuts. They don't do as well with processed sugars, processed grains, and low-fat dairy products.

Types of Fire in the Body

What is fire in the body? Obviously there aren't any little flames burning hither and dither throughout our cells. Or are there? Using our basic definition of fire as an oxidative process, let's think about the oxidative processes in our bodies. Sometimes these processes are called redox reactions when the process applies to elements other than oxygen.

First and foremost, digestion is an oxidative process, though a slow one in comparison to a blazing fire. During digestion, the food that we eat containing fats, carbohydrates, and proteins makes its way through different parts of the gastrointestinal tract. Each part of the digestive tract has its own specific environment. Food is first exposed to the enzymes in the saliva in the mouth, then the acid-based gastric juices in the stomach, then digestive enzymes and bile in the small intestine, and, last, the fermenting anaerobic bacteria of the large intestine. Each part of the digestive system has its own environment and its own role in the oxidative processes of digestion. Just like fire leaves ash in its wake, digestion leaves wastes that are excreted through feces and urine.

Another oxidative process (fire) in the body is the production of raw energy. For many of us, when we think of energy, we think about the raw energy that we need to play sports, go to work, or putter around the house. That certainly is a valid type of energy related to blood sugar that we tend to manipulate throughout the day with sugar and caffeine.

But there is another type of energy—cellular energy. Our cells and organ systems require a continuous supply of energy to maintain the healthy functioning of our bodies. Every second throughout the day, our bodies are busy performing all the functions vital to our existence. While we are sleeping, our bodies are busy repairing tissue, building bones, fighting infections, and processing toxins. Where does that cellular energy come from?

To create cellular energy, our bodies take nutrients from food and produce ATP, or adenosine triphosphate. The production of ATP is another type of fire that is taking place within our cells using oxidation-reduction reactions. Without ATP, we wouldn't be alive. Influencing factors on cellular energy production include nutrient intake, mitochondria health, and thyroid activity level. Creating cellular energy, creating good fire, is a three-stage process.

First, during digestion, using an oxidative process, food has to be broken down by enzymes into a form that can be used by the mitochondria, the powerhouses of the cells. Proteins have to be broken down into amino acids; complex carbohydrates into sugars; and fats into fatty acids and glycerol. Once nutrients are broken down into their smallest and simplest forms, they are taken to the cells, where they gradually oxidize in energy production.

In the second stage of energy production, glucose is broken down into pyruvate which is taken up by the mitochondria within each cell. And in the third stage, mitochondria, using the nutrients from food, creates our main energy, ATP.

The ash produced from ATP production is free radicals, which can damage our mitochondria, clog cells, and reduce our energy and feelings of well-being. Extensive oxidative damage has been implicated in type 2 diabetes, Alzheimer's disease, autoimmune disorders, and inflammatory disorders. It's also been implicated in how long we live. When our mitochondria are damaged, we suffer. Our physical and mental energy levels drop, and our Vital Energy level drops as well. Importantly, when mitochondria are injured, they release a chemical that triggers cell death. Yikes! Ultimately, you want to keep these little powerhouses as healthy as possible by eating foods that are high in antioxidant nutrients, exercising on a regular basis, and getting good-quality sleep. Antioxidants include vitamins A, C, E, selenium, and the phytonutrients resveratrol and lutein.

So much of what we consider our cellular energy or vitality, our Vital Energy, boils down to what's happening within the cell with the mitochondria. Remember the mitochondrial DNA we inherit from our mothers? Well here it is at work creating our Vital Energy. What is Vital Energy anyway? It is the energy of our life force. It fuels our passion, drive, creativity, motivation, and good health. Vital Energy is our good fire and helps us recover after illness and bounce back after emotional trauma. Every constitution, when in balance, has good Vital Energy because every constitution is sparked by the oxidative processes of energy production via mitochondria within the cell.

Just a little rabbit trail: Mitochondria are interesting little creatures. They are more closely related to bacteria than to us. All life on earth, from humans to animals to plants, has a symbiotic relationship with mitochondria; we can't live without them and they can't live without us. We are in a fixed and permanent relationship with these creatures that aren't us but live inside each of our individual cells. Mitochondria contain their own DNA, which we inherit from our mothers, known as mitochondrial DNA (mtDNA), which we discussed in an earlier chapter. Thinking about the fact that we inherit our mitochondrial DNA from our mothers and their primary function is energy production, it is quite easy to extrapolate that the baseline of our Vital Energy is directly inherited from our mothers. Of course, there are other influences on our Vital Energy to consider such as diet, overall genetics, environment, and lifestyle choices.

And all this begins with digestion.

Other fire or oxidative processes in the body include purine metabolism, the conversion of long-chain fatty acids into medium-chain fatty acids, inflammation, the ingestion of bacteria by infection fighters, the metabolism of arachidonic acid, the act of physical movement and exercise, phase 1 detoxification in the liver, and the tissue damage caused by reduced blood supply to an area.

Lifestyle choices and environment can also initiate oxidative processes that create free radicals including cigarette smoking, environmental pollutants, radiation exposure, certain prescription medications, pesticides, industrial solvents, and ozone. In today's polluted world, it's never a bad idea to supplement with a good antioxidant formula.

The Fire Is in the Fat

Fire is associated with the body fluid or humor of bile, which is yellow, and the taste of bitter. Have you ever been really sick and throwing up, and you keep vomiting until there's nothing left in your stomach? Then, when you think you can't throw up anymore, here comes this disgusting, bitter yellow liquid. That is bile.

Bile has the significant function of emulsifying fats in the digestive process. To understand the nature of the fire element, it is important to understand the process of fat digestion, the nature of bile, and the taste of bitter. Bile is manufactured in the liver and stored and released by the gallbladder to aid in the digestion of fats. It emulsifies fat into smaller and smaller particles so that the enzyme lipase can convert the fat into fatty acids in an oxidative process. These are then carried to the cells by the lymphatic system or moved into storage through the bloodstream.

Fatty acids are the preferred fuel for fire folk in the ATP process, also known as cellular respiration, citric acid cycle, and Krebs cycle. You know the process must be important if it has three different names. Normally, glucose is the preferred fuel for producing energy; it's quick, cheap, and readily available. Just grab another doughnut. But using simple carbohydrates as energy has drawbacks such as elevated blood sugar, weight gain, and crashing once the sugar is gone.

Actually, the mitochondria can use carbohydrates, fats, or proteins for fuel, the latter two with a little conversion. The body will only use protein if it is absolutely necessary and no other fuel is available, but would prefer to use carbohydrates or fats. The byproduct of breaking down protein is ammonia. It stands to reason that folks on a high-protein, low-carbohydrate diet will produce more ammonia than someone on a more balanced diet. Ammonia has to be excreted by the kidneys, which is why high-protein diets strain the kidneys. If there aren't enough dietary nutrients available, the body will use protein for fuel in the form of muscle breakdown. This will cause the muscle wasting that is often found after a long illness or in wasting diseases.

Using fatty acids for fuel is a cleaner burn and isn't quick, cheap, and easy. Fatty acids must be converted and combined with coenzyme A to feed into the Krebs cycle. Fire folks will gravitate toward fats and often decline desserts, preferring salty and fatty to sweet and fatty. Also eating too much fat can also cause weight gain with fire people, while eating excess carbohydrates is the main culprit with the other constitutions.

Because we need fat, we need bile, and because we need bile, we need bitter foods and herbs, which help release the flow of bile from our gallbladder or encourage its production in the liver. Common bitter herbs to aid fat digestion include dandelion, gentian, milk thistle, blessed thistle, American ginseng, hops, yarrow, and peppermint. A bitter salad with a meal will also improve fat digestion.

In general, folks with a dominant fire element like to eat fat; it is soothing and comforting for body and soul. They will eat the well-cooked fat from the steak or double the amount of olive oil in the salad dressing. Fire folks can demolish a half-stick of butter with a meal, especially if feeling stressed, and nary experience a rise in cholesterol levels. The quality of the fat is extremely important, and wild game or pasture-raised meats are vitally necessary for healthy fire and are good sources of omega oils. Fire folk should be cautious with a grain-based diet lacking in adequate protein and fat, as this will definitely contribute to weight gain, even with exercise.

Active fire people tend to burn fat rather than store it. An overweight fire person is truly out of balance and more than likely not moving or exercising enough. Without movement, there is also a tendency toward constipation, which adds to the appearance of weight gain around the center gut area and hips because fire folk are prone to inflamed small intestines and other digestive difficulties. Often their constipation is related to lack of movement of food through the small intestines, not the large intestine or colon. The partially digested food builds and builds in the small intestines creating inflammation, leaky gut syndrome, constipation, and poor metabolism of nutrients; this is often related to lack of movement in general. This can also apply to the air constitution, or sour blood. Like fire moving across the land, fire people need to move to be healthy and generally love exercise of any type, but especially competitive activities. When fire people don't move, their energy drops to a smolder instead of a steady burn.

The Bitter Taste of Bile

The taste of bile is bitter and rises in the back of the throat. It's no accident that the majority of bitter taste buds can be found primarily on the back of the tongue, the roof of the mouth, and on the soft palate. But do keep in mind that all four different taste buds are found all over the tongue; bitter is just slightly clustered toward the back.

Bitter is the taste that protects us from poisonous plants and foods since many poisonous alkaloids are bitter-tasting. Just take a bite of something really bitter and see what happens. The reflexive reaction is to shake the head with the eyes shut and stick out the tongue and drool. Your body has stopped the swallowing process and has initiated the spitting process to stop you from swallowing the bitter poison. How long do you drool and spit after tasting extreme bitterness?

I will venture to say that balanced fire folk have well-developed tastes of bitter and don't mind the bitter taste in herbs and vegetable sources. Deficient fire folk might be overly sensitive to the bitter taste, while excess fire might crave it and reach for the broccoli instead of the potato, simply because they are eating more fats. Tannins found in many herbs and in black tea taste bitter. Coffee has a bitter taste.

The taste of bitter initiates bile flow, which helps facilitate a bowel movement. Fat will also initiate the flow of bile and help facilitate a bowel movement. Don't be surprised to find that a fire person does their morning business after a cup of coffee or tea and sausage or bacon, or some other fatty food. Carbohydrates for breakfast just cause poor energy and morning constipation. Bitter herbs for digestion include yellow dock, wild yam, blue vervain, milk thistle, gentian, and dandelion.

Some people have bile reflux (excess fire), with symptoms similar to that of heartburn (also excess fire). Bile reflux is due to a backup of bile and digestive fluids that should have stayed in the small intestine but are now in the stomach. It is often mistakenly diagnosed as acid reflux, though this may also be present. Bile reflux can cause discomfort or a burning sensation in the lower esophagus, but more noticeably in the stomach due to resulting inflammation in the lining. It requires immediate attention to avoid ulcerations in these tissues.

Bile is so alkaline that it burns. Soap makers who have worked with lye, another strong alkaline, will understand the reference. In the soap-making process, when you're pouring the lye into the water, the bowl will literally get hot to touch. The alkaline lye is all the heat that is needed to "cook" the soap. So it is with bile. This extreme alkalinity is very caustic to the mucous membrane tissues. Bile may be present in stools in cases of extreme diarrhea, gallbladder problems, irritable bowel syndrome, flu, or food poisoning. Bile may also be present in stools after doing a "gallbladder cleanse," and the excess release of bile is often confused with passing gallstones or passing toxins.

Water is the element that reduces the heat of bile and puts out fire. It is the initial treatment for any caustic alkaline burn, whether in the body or in the laboratory. Water applied quickly, either physically or metaphorically, reduces the damage of excessive fire, but won't address the cause of it. Air will fan the flames and can fuel it or blow it out of control. Earth can smother fire or cause a bad burn with the wrong fuel.

Salt neutralizes the taste of bitter. The ions in the salt block the receptors that taste bitter, a neat little chemical reaction. That's why a little salt in your coffee will eliminate any bitterness. For fire people, salt helps control the fire, control the bitter. Salt is the opposite taste of bitter, and water is the opposite element. This is a handy tip to keep in mind.

Salt also helps control histamine levels and fire folks are prone to high histamine, which may manifest as food allergies, seasonal allergies, rashes, swollen eyes and legs, and hives. You might notice that fire folk aren't stingy with the salt shaker either, and will tend to salt their food without even tasting it.

Without adequate intake of water and fat, fire people have dry skin and hair and digestive and kidney issues. They must discern if dryness is due to lack of oil or lack of water. Fire folk on an extremely low-fat diet suffer tremendously. They may experience dry skin, hair, and nails, reproductive dysfunction, low energy and fatigue, and lack of motivation and creativity. Add a little fat to the diet and it all comes back.

When fire is low and energy is down, fire people may also crave the taste of sour, which is the element air. Any good fire needs a steady supply of oxygen or it will go out. For this reason, fire folk often need to nourish their fire with air by eating sour foods. For example, lemon water upon rising can help start digestion for the day. Fire people may also enjoy fermented foods, but prefer the sourness of fermented vegetables and pickles to that of fermented dairy.

Fire people tend to exhibit higher than normal rates of total cholesterol on standard blood tests. Always check the ratio between HDL and LDL components on your blood work. If the ratios are good, and they often are with good levels of HDL, then address your doctor's concerns with information about ratios instead of overall total numbers. If the ratios between HDL and LDL aren't considered good, then you may have some work to do. Often increasing good fats, such as omega-3 fish oils, and exercising is all that's needed to bring those ratios in line.

As the characteristics of fire people are explored in the following section, think about the nature and interaction of fire, bile, and fat. Fire cannot exist alone; it must have fuel. Fuel for the human body is preferably either carbohydrates or fat. Fat needs bile to be metabolized. Because bile is produced in the liver and stored and released from the gallbladder, fire people must nurture these organs for good health. And fire people must protect and nurture their hearts both physically and metaphorically.

Influence of Fire

The fire element influences the head, brain, heart, spine, eyes, upper back, hips, thighs, gallbladder, and liver. It governs and is enhanced by metabolism and mitochondrial energy production, as well as thyroid and pancreas activity levels.

Fire is also involved in the production of prostaglandins and other fat-based inflammatory factors, stress hormones such as epinephrine and norepinephrine, and reproductive hormones such as estrogen and testosterone. If fat is involved in the function, just think fire.

Functions of the liver related to phase 1 and 2 detoxification, methylation, and hormone metabolism fall under the domain of fire. The liver is our natural detoxification organ, getting rid of water-soluble toxins in phase 1 and fat-soluble toxins, alcohol, prescription medications, and environmental toxins in phase 2. Herbs that support the detox function of the liver include milk thistle, blessed thistle, burdock, fenugreek, fennel, cayenne, and peppermint. These same herbs support the methylation process, which also helps remove toxins from our bodies, repair DNA, and affect epigenetics. Hormone conversion or metabolism also takes place in the liver. For example, T4 produced by the thyroid must be converted to T3, the useable form, and then sent to the cells. This conversion takes place in the liver.

Inflammation, chronic or acute, creates oxidation that damages tissues. Chronic inflammation plays a role in a wide variety of age-related disorders including diabetes, cardiovascular disease, chronic digestive difficulties, and autoimmune disorders and may speed the aging process. The oxidative stress that occurs during the inflammatory processes uses vast amounts of antioxidant nutrients to offset the number of free radicals produced. If the number of free radicals overwhelms the amount of available antioxidants, then the fatty acids and proteins within the cell membrane may be permanently damaged, which will affect the functioning of the cell. In addition, excess free radicals can lead to cell mutation and DNA damage which can be a risk for cancers and other disorders. Again, antioxidant nutrients include vitamins A, C, E, selenium, and the phytonutrients resveratrol and lutein.

Hives, rashes, swellings, histamine reactions, redness after insect bites, and other signs of inflammation speak of fire. Joint swellings that are warm to touch or red fall under fire's domain. Fever, sunburn, infection with fever, heat, or redness also speak to fire.

Two of our most important organs—the brain and the heart—fall under the domain of fire. The brain is composed of fatty acids but burns glucose; the heart burns fatty acids. Healthy fats and their proper digestion and assimilation are exceptionally important to fire people. This helps keep them physically healthy and emotionally balanced.

The eyes, upper back, hips, and thighs are muscle systems that are involved in our fight-or-flight response and many athletic activities. Fire folk make good competitive athletes and fit warriors who derive a great amount of enjoyment and stress relief through physical activity. Active fire people have a well-trained cerebellum, the part of the brain that is located in the back of the skull that coordinates physical activity and muscular coordination. The cerebellum also is responsible for the hand-eye coordination that is required for athletic activity.

Fire Traits

People with a dominant fire element are passionate, creative, competitive, courageous, honorable, enthusiastic, intelligent, individualist, and strong-willed. Fire people have high energy levels and strong Vital Energy. They are extroverted, funny, honest, and independent. They tend to be explorers, whether of land or mind, and love learning new things and putting things together in new and different ways.

Dopamine is the neurotransmitter associated with fire because it helps fuel exploration, curiosity, and risk-taking, and helps create the memory of the exploration. Add a little testosterone and think of the fiery Celts who explored new lands, pillaging along the way, but never creating settlements or strong systems of government, and you get the picture.

Fire folk tend to be charismatic, and by the force and fire of their personality, these people can draw others to them. Politicians often have strong fire in their constitution, especially the ones that exhibit the most charisma. Actors and actresses, entertainers, and singers often lure us into their orbit because of the sheer force of their personalities. Fire people also make good commanding officers who automatically receive loyalty and devotion from their troops.

They often yearn for a great work in life—their great commitment. Their goals and projects are where fire people put their energy and drive. Their work or projects are the center of their lives, the reason to get up every morning. They expect those they love, family or friends, to support their work and projects just as much as they do themselves. It's taken very personally when support isn't shown to their satisfaction. These are the folks who define themselves through their work or interests.

Fire people are loyal and make friends and mates for life unless there is mass betrayal in the relationship. However, their closest friends are generally those found through their work. These are the people with similar interests that draw flame to flame. The fire person will also dote on those friends who are willing to step forward in the face of adversity and support the fire person. This sort of comradery, this willingness to step forward, is appreciated and never forgotten.

Their competitive nature and curious mind spurs them to learn a great deal of information about a variety of subjects. This is not a shallow knowing; they can generally use all the information they have accumulated for their projects, events, tasks, or goals. They make great inventors, creative people on projects, college professors, and good public speakers. Fire people love to share what they know.

The people with a dominant fire element are driven to spread themselves thin, much as fire spreads across the land. As long as there is a job or project to drive them, they will burn with a consuming passion. Problems arise when they take on too many projects at one time. They will work at their projects or jobs long hours, often to the detriment of their health and their personal lives. There is great honor and satisfaction in completing their task and of a job well done. This doesn't necessarily equate to happiness, but at least to satisfaction and an increase in self-esteem. A caution for fire people—too many irons in the fire can lead to burnout.

Fire people are seldom depressed, and when they are feeling low, it doesn't last very long. They are generally fun and sunny people who try to find quick solutions to problems that arise either in their work, projects, or personal lives.

Fire people need movement to be healthy. Exercise is invigorating and rejuvenating to these folks, balances blood sugar, and oxygenates the body. In the same way that a fire needs oxygen to burn brightly, so do fire people, and exercise and deep breathing help. Fire folk can actually get more energy by going for a walk than from a cup of coffee.

As long as fire people eat nutritiously (fuel) and move (air), and don't take on too many projects, they will maintain a healthy weight, produce high Vital Energy, and live to an old age. And as long as fire people move and exercise, they can handle tremendous amounts of stress, especially the stress that is generated by their own constant projects, or the stress that is generated when family and friends want more time and attention than the fire person can spare from the job or project.

When fire doesn't move, when fire people sit too long, blood and lymph slows, and pretty soon they gain weight and digestion becomes sluggish. There is also fatigue, loss of drive and motivation, and a soft, bloated look. If this scenario continues, the fire person will begin to take on some traits from their opposite, water.

Fire folk generally have well-defined muscles and medium-width bones. Muscle definition doesn't mean bulky muscles; it simply means well-toned muscles. A fire person may not exercise for months and when they restart their program, muscle tone and definition return in a very short time. Suddenly calves will appear defined, the muscle area around the knee will be defined, and arms will also. The more a fire person exercises, the more defined the large muscles become; and this includes the heart.

Protein and fat are better breakfast choices to start the day than carbohydrates. Oatmeal for breakfast without added protein is sure to mess with the blood sugar for the morning, if not the rest of the day. Carbohydrates for breakfast only makes the fire person sleepy, groggy, and operating under brain fog. A quick nap is needed to right this situation, and then a meal with protein, fat, and complex carbohydrates.

Fire people love children, their own and other people's, and they like pets. Unfortunately, they are often too busy with their work and projects to give either children or pets the full attention that might be needed. Unless of course being a parent is their job and then, look out, they are supreme.

These folks are intuitive by nature and occasionally appear psychic. Their innate intuition allows them to see patterns that others don't and to extrapolate quickly and efficiently. This is a handy talent that provides creative input for their projects or work.

One of the characteristics of fire is that it transforms. Vulcan, the god of the forge, transformed rock into metal. Fire folks can take an idea and totally transform it into something new and innovative. They don't mind bucking convention either.

Fire people seek a supportive partner, someone who understands and appreciates their talents and what they can accomplish. With the right supporting relationship or business partner, there's no limit to what a fire person can do. Fire folk often have multiple marriages or love affairs looking for that right partner. In truth, fire burns the brightest with the right mix of air, fuel (earth), and moisture—and so does the fire constitution.

Think of Will and Ariel Durant. Will was a philosopher, writer, and historian who over his career published hundreds of books and magazine articles, and with his wife, Ariel, wrote the classic *The Story of Civilization* in eleven volumes. Together they were an amazing team. Will was the fire and Ariel the supporting earth. They both lived well into their nineties, died within weeks of each other, but had no children. Other examples of such couples are Amelia Earhart and George Putnam; Marie and Pierre Curie; the Reverend Martin Luther King, Jr., and Coretta Scott King; Franklin Delano and Eleanor Roosevelt; and Diego Rivera and Frida Kahlo.

Fire folk often create their personal identity around what they do or their profession. This can create self-esteem issues if they lose their job, their project is a failure, or their profession goes through great changes. Interestingly, fire people may have several different professions over their life span, each one creating a personal identification and self-esteem value. These are the folks who should never retire; it can bring too much loss of identity.

Remember, we all have some fire.

Excess Fire

Excess fire is easy to identify: Anger, anger, and more anger. The anger is always just below the surface waiting to erupt. Stress, perceived personal slights, losing a job, trauma, feeling betrayed, or illness can be the culprit. Often, the anger stems from childhood bullying, especially in junior high school, or other childhood trauma that has been suppressed but smoldering for years until something triggers it. Self-esteem issues are dominant. It may also show in the personality as temper, impatience, and being overly critical. Any little thing will set off the eruption of unresolved anger that lies just below the surface. Excess fire will also show in controlling behavior, and rigidity and inflexibility when making decisions. When fire is in excess, the person must attempt to control the blaze or it becomes a forest fire, out of control.

Folks will lose their normal spontaneity and creativity. Peripheral mental vision is lost, the blinders go on, and work becomes a stress and chore. Control issues emerge.

There are almost always too many irons in the fire from taking on too many new projects or creative endeavors simultaneously. Somehow, the fire person feels that if they take on more projects, somehow, this will smooth things out, when actually the opposite is happening.

People with excess fire tend to lash out at the ones they love the most when under stress. The ego dominates and fire pulls into protective mode. Unfortunately, in extreme situations, the anger fuels physical violence. It was a well-known fact that before air conditioning, the murder rate soared during the summer months in the South. The heat is irritating to every system in the body, especially the nerves, and anger is just as irritating on the nervous system.

Other signs of excess fire are nervousness, hyperalertness, anxiety and/or irritability, heart palpitations, trouble sleeping, tremor, muscle weakness, digestive disturbances, sweating, weight loss even though eating, heat intolerance, and reproductive dysfunction. Other signs of excess fire can include anxiety, restlessness, fidgeting, chewing the fingernails, very fine, silky hair without body, tremor of fingers and tongue, rapid speech, increased blood pressure, thirst, and overall dryness.

Excess fire may exhibit as thick blood, fever, inflammation, and rashes. High blood pressure, stroke, heart attack, and cardiovascular disease can also result from excessive fire that has thickened the blood. Excess fire can cause dehydration and loss of fluid, which is a contributing factor. In hyperthyroidism, the body will literally burn itself up. Infection is an obvious source of fire as the immune system fights against invaders. In excess fire, the face tends toward redness, as do the fingernails. The tongue may also be red and irritated-looking or have a red tip.

When under stress, the fire initially flames, and folks tend to reach for the salty, fatty potato chips and nuts rather than the chocolate chip cookies to support the fire needed to complete their project or reach the finish line. Maintaining excess fire can take a severe toll on the body, mind, and spirit as the fire burns through vast amounts of nutrients, creates excessive free radicals, and damages mitochondria and the endocrine system. The damage to the endocrine system can result in hypothyroidism, type 2 diabetes, and adrenal exhaustion. This situation will move the person from excessive fire to deficient fire.

Cooling, moist herbs and foods and plenty of fluids help bring excess fire back toward balance. These foods and herbs also tend to contain minerals that help regulate the Krebs cycle, nervous system, and endocrine system. Cooling foods include moist fruits and berries, which are chock-full of antioxidants: greens, Navy beans, green beans, seafood, fresh cheeses, yogurt, melons, cucumbers, Great Northern beans, lima beans, lentils, and green peppers.

Cooling herbs include sumac, dill, yarrow, elder flower, lemon balm, lemon verbena, peppermint, boneset, chamomile, blessed thistle, Monarda, sage, corn silk, skullcap, bilberry, dandelion, bugleweed, plantain, catnip, slippery elm, spearmint, hydrangea, marshmallow, and yucca. It's important to determine if cooling, moistening herbs are needed or if cooling, drying herbs are needed, and this will depend upon the given situation.

It's also a good idea to reduce fat intake when fire is in excess, especially animal fat from mammals. At the same time, an increase in omega-3 fatty acids from fish and sea vegetables can help cool the body and reduce inflammation. Animal fat is heating and only adds fuel to an already blazing fire.

Deficient Fire

A person with low fire lacks passion, cries easily, and feels very sorry for themselves. A deficient fire person will exhibit many traits in common with the water person, which is fire's opposite. When fire is low, the personality has a true tendency toward bitterness, self-pity, and depression. During this time of low fire, folks cling to unhealthy relationships and feel that life has no meaning or that things will never change. They also tend to feel unsupported and alone.

In deficient fire, people feel overwhelmed and overextended. When fire is low, energy is low and creativity is down. Self-preservation and survival are the goal, whether physical or emotional. The thought of changing the situation doesn't cross the mind because folks are in survival mode. When the idea of changing the situation is mentioned as an option or remedy for the situation, the fire person will stare with incredulity that change is even suggested. Talk about thinking in a rut! Everything just seems hopeless. This is the time when fire needs the support of family and friends, stimulating herbs, spices and foods, mild, bitter diuretics, and a return to a fire-supporting diet with reduced grains.

It would seem that the fire person would reach for good fats and proteins in this situation, but the opposite tends to happen. When energy is reduced, the fire person tends to gravitate toward simple carbohydrates, looking for quick energy. The person who never wanted dessert now has a dessert at every meal, and snacks too. The person that was happy with fruit as a sweet now wants to eat cakes, pies, and cookies. The person who used honey for a sweetener and avoided processed sugar now grabs the sugar jar. Carbohydrates are a quick energy source that lifts energy for a short time, but then suddenly drops it like a hot potato. In no time at all, more carbohydrates are needed to get the energy up and going.

The classic example of deficient fire disorder is hypothyroidism. Energy is low, fatigue is common, nutrient uptake is limited, circulation is sluggish, there is disturbed digestion, low functioning of all major organs, lymph is stagnant, and the body becomes cool and watery. There is reduced drive and passion for life, low motivation, and almost nonexistent creativity. All this is a perfect breeding ground for parasites, both physical and psychic. And the low fire person feels very victimized.

Common signs of deficient fire may include fatigue, lethargy, cold intolerance, weight gain, digestive difficulties, edema, arthritis-type pain, nerve pain, diminished libido, infertility, menstrual problems, headache, low blood sugar, slow thinking, confusion, clumsiness, constipation, slow stomach emptying, rashes, poor immune functioning, recurrent infections, lymphatic congestion, loss of muscle strength, depression, low blood pressure, elevated cholesterol, anemia, and liver difficulties.

Other signs of deficient fire might include a round, puffy face, a large, swollen tongue, large or swollen hands, lack of muscle tone, loose joints, muscle weakness, delayed reflexes, yellowish skin, scaling, dry skin, cool skin, dry nails, enlarged or overworked heart, low core temperature, skin tags, lack of sweating, dry, brittle nails, and slow speech.

A deficiency of fire can present as cool blood, which is thin, weak, and watery, with low pressure. Anemia may be present. There is stagnation and swelling in the abdomen and low flow of body fluids, including bile and lymph. The face tends to be pale, as do the nails, and there may be dark circles under the eyes. The skin loses its luster and takes on a yellowish tint. Digestion is sluggish and assimilation of nutrients is poor. The bowels may be sluggish, and congestion may be present in the lungs and around the heart. Mucus tends to gather in any and all mucous membrane tissues but doesn't move. Vital Energy is low, movement is an effort, and the heart beats with a strain. There is a tendency to hold fluid in the abdomen, breasts, buttocks, and upper thighs. Stimulation is desperately needed.

Warming foods and herbs can help build a sustained fire. These include soups and stews, animal protein, onions, garlic, winter squashes, pumpkin, summer squashes, cooked greens, butter, olive oil, potatoes, sweet potatoes, yam, kidney beans, black beans, and seaweeds.

Warming and/or stimulating herbs include cayenne, milk thistle, American ginseng, blessed thistle, red clover, black pepper, peppermint, cinnamon, cloves, angelica, kelp, licorice, pine, lobelia, sarsaparilla, horseradish, bay, and sassafras.

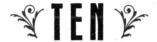 TEN

Water: Salty Blood

My fake plants died because I did not pretend to water them.
—Mitch Hedberg

OVER HER WORKING CAREER, Mama worked outside the cotton fields in three different professions, each of them hard on the body. She worked as a cook, which wasn't physically as hard as field work but in some ways was more stressful because she had to deal with the public and had to keep them satisfied and happy with her cooking. Mama was considered a good Southern cook and could plan the menu for and feed about fifty people a meat and three vegetables, cornbread, sweet tea, and dessert five days a week at the local café. To this day, diners and cafes are my favorite places to eat either in town or on the road, and I look for these small, family-run businesses wherever I travel. The food is generally decent and filling, and it brings me great comfort to be in the environment I know so well, a part of my upbringing, and a touch of home on the road. Wherever Mama worked, us kids always visited, and we became almost as familiar with the setting as she was.

Mama worked as a cook during the off-times from the cotton fields, and then later, after the cotton-picking jobs were given to mechanical harvesters, she cooked full time. Papa Bright, like many tenant farmers, was forced by his landlords to rent mechanical cotton harvesters because it was cheaper than paying for human labor. Both my Mama and her sister Sadie went to work as cooks. Sadie eventually got a job in the textiles making blue jeans, but not Mama.

Mama also cleaned houses for a living. It didn't pay any better than cooking, but the hours were better. Most families didn't want her to start until 8 a.m., and she worked until their kids came home from school, though occasionally she stayed and cooked supper for the family before coming home and doing the same for us. Huntsville, Alabama, had seen a great influx of highly educated people from other states coming to work for NASA or for the government in some capacity such as missile development in the defense industry. Many of these transplants moved to outlying small towns, trading the commute to work for cheap land. In a very short time, our area went from a farming community to a bedroom community, and life changed forever.

With the influx of so many new people, all professions of the middle class grew; we suddenly had doctors, lawyers, dentists, and pharmacists. Not that we didn't have doctors before; we had two. And the town had a couple of lawyers and a dentist. But now, with population growth, we had several of each. The town was certainly changing.

All the newcomers had funny accents, called Yankee by most locals. The newcomers found they could hire help to clean their houses, raise their kids, and do their yard work and handiwork for very little of nothing. These transplants set themselves up to remake the town to be similar to the ones they had left behind, which occasionally caused rifts and troubles among them and the town's local population. It certainly forced some progress on the town.

One benefit of the outsiders moving to town was that our school system immediately improved. The children joining our schools found themselves two or three grades ahead of where we locals were at the same age. So a third-grade girl moving from Michigan found herself in the fifth grade here. Because of the dedicated efforts of the transplants, our town now has one of the best public school systems in the state.

With the improved economy, Mama found a niche as a housekeeper and sometimes a nanny, a task that she excelled at doing the same way she had excelled at cotton picking. She once said to me, "When I leave a clean house at the end of the day, I know I've made a difference in those people's lives." And she believed this with her whole heart and soul. She felt sorry for those children who depended upon a stranger to make their beds, cook their food, and soothe their feverish brows while their own mamas were off playing bridge, at a club meeting, or shopping. Mama repeatedly told us how lucky we were that she was teaching us to take care of ourselves, that we were learning how to run our own homes when we got married. "Be independent," she'd say, "take care of yourself." We, however, looked at the nice clothes, nice houses, and new cars of the better-off families and wondered whether independence and housekeeping skills were an even trade-off. Today, I understand and appreciate how she taught us to take care of ourselves, especially when I look at the younger generations raised without the cooking, shopping, banking, cleaning, and life skills that we all need to navigate adulthood.

Before the transplants came to town, there were only two classes of people: the haves and the have-nots. The haves were people who owned land or a business and had money, which often had been passed down through the family (affectionately called "old money"). The have-nots were everyone else. It was a system that had been in place for generations and there was resistance to change, even among the have-nots.

Now suddenly there was a third category. The people that were well-educated and made good money working in the space or defense industry. These folks didn't fit into the social scheme and didn't care. Most of them came from regular working-class families in their home states but had aspired to something different by way of an education in the sciences. Education changed everything. Locals could now see the results of what a good education could bring regardless of your family's money status or who your people were. A good education could pay off.

Sometimes Mama brought home hand-me-down clothes given to her by one of the ladies of the houses she cleaned. These beautiful clothes were a huge change from either the hand-me-downs of cousins or the clothes Mama made for us, which used the same pattern and style over and over that was at least twenty years out of date. Store-bought clothes were reserved for special items such as coats and underwear and socks and shoes. Mama was an excellent seamstress, and one year she was hired to sew the high school cheerleading uniforms.

One time, Mama brought home two big boxes of beautiful clothes. I had never seen such fine material or stylish clothes and even I, at a time when I really had no idea of the cost of bought things, knew that these clothes were expensive. The material just felt soft and lovely, not like the material of my homemade clothes that were a bit rough on the skin until washed at least a dozen times. The clothes all fit me like a glove and were my favorite colors. I went to school floating on a cloud. Two days later the clothes were gone. Disappeared from my closet and nowhere to be found. Mama had given them away. After the shock and disappointment wore off, I asked her through my tears why she had done that. "They gave you airs," was all she said. Back to my old, worn hand-me-downs and out-of-date clothes.

I understand that Mama was trying to protect me. Wearing nice store-bought clothes gave the appearance of money we didn't have. Here I was, dressed really nice, and my siblings weren't. It was an inequality that I'm not even sure she had the words to explain. She was also afraid that having nice store-bought things might set the yearning for more, a yearning that couldn't be fulfilled by our family and that would just lead to unhappiness. From her point of view, I would grow up to sew in a factory, work in a plant, or maybe, if lucky, be a teacher or secretary. Those were all good professions for a young lady, and that was success. But I wanted something different. And me wanting something different set the stage for strife in our relationship for many years to come. Even after I became successful enough as an herbalist to buy a house, she asked, "Why don't you get some steady work and quit all that herb stuff?"

Our town had a small boom and suddenly factories were built. Mama left cleaning houses and caring for other people's children behind and got a job cleaning bathrooms in a factory. She was more than pleased; she was proud of being the janitor for the plant. Mama finally had a job that paid Social Security and a bit of retirement. She was making twice the money she made cleaning houses, worked shorter hours, and got a full lunch break. Mama loved socializing with the other workers and made many friends in the plant. Now she had two communities, church and work. Although all the years of hard work and struggling to make ends meet and feed her family took a toll on her health and her body, she managed to keep the position until she turned sixty-five and could retire. Even after she retired, Mama would go back to the plant and visit with the friends she had made. Unfortunately, the plant closed and moved to Mexico with the NAFTA agreement, as did many of the other plants in town, leaving hundreds of people scrambling for jobs without the benefit of cotton fields to return to and a lot of big empty buildings.

Mama worked hard her whole life; nothing seemed to come easy for her or our family. Her faith and belief guided her through great difficulties, especially the years after my father strayed and then left us. During those lean years, we were so poor that once Mama sold our beds to pay the electric bill. She never let go her belief, her relationship to God, or her relationship to her fellow church members. For Mama, these were the most important relationships.

I think that mother/daughter relationships are the most challenging to navigate, and Mama and I certainly found this to be true. She firmly believed that life should be lived according to the Bible and didn't deter from that belief, in thought or action, her whole life. My mama had faith, and it never wavered. I was rebellious, creative, and wanted something different from my life. At age fifteen, I took the scissors and chopped my hair to pieces. It had never been cut due to religious reasons, and this was a blow to her very heart. She cried for days but eventually carried me to a hair dresser to make my hair look more presentable because I had chopped it terribly. This was the beginning of many years of unhealthy actions and a strained relationship between us.

Over the course of my adult life, however strained our relationship, Mama was always there whenever I needed her. I never had any doubt of that fact nor of her love for me. Like many people, I really didn't know my mother well until right before she died. During our conversations in her final months, I found out that she had wanted to study business law but felt her religion prevented that. Business law? Who wants to study business law? But Mama did. She also disclosed that she had wanted to travel and see some of the famous gardens across the South, but thought that might be wrong too. She had been taught to stay home and keep the land and house, and that she did. I found out that she had been engaged before she married my father, but that man had died in a motorcycle accident and she was the one that identified his body. I found out that after Mama and Daddy got married, that it took two years for her to get pregnant and she was so happy and excited to be a mother that she paraded around town with her growing belly in a time when pregnant women were supposed to stay home and not be seen. I found out that she was two years old before her parents named her because they weren't sure she was going to live. They called her "Baby Girl." It was a neighbor that finally named her: Esther Pauline.

My mother was all about relationships, belief, and faith—a true water person. The most important relationship in Mama's life was her relationship with God. She spent her whole life living to go to heaven. Every decision she made, every opinion she gave, every thought or action was centered around her relationship with God. Mama believed. Next, was her relationship with my father. Even though they were separated for ten years and then reunited, she never wavered in her love for him. At Daddy's funeral, my brothers had to drag her away from the coffin in tears, her body stiff with grief. She couldn't stand to lose him. Mama's relationship with her children came next in her life, and then, later, her grandchildren.

If you went to her for advice, Mama didn't hesitate to give you the direct, straight truth of what she saw without any sugar coating. Sometimes this was tough to hear, but sometimes it was exactly what you needed. But Mama wasn't only water; there was fire there also. In high school, she was put in detention for fighting more than once. Mama had a terrible temper that flared unexpectedly when you least expected it. She had a fiery passion for her beliefs that went beyond mere relationship. Her beliefs were her project, her reason for living. I miss her terribly.

Mama believed in love though its waters may not have always dampened her feet the way she would have liked. From Song of Solomon, "Many waters cannot quench love, neither can floods drown it. If a man offered for love all the wealth of his house, he would be utterly despised." This one's for you Mama.

All About Water

First and foremost: Water is wet. I know that sounds obvious, but it needed stating. The temperature of water is dependent upon whether it is being heated or cooled. Both water and earth are heated by radiation from the sun and by the transfer of heat from the Earth's core. In our body, the water, our fluids, are heated by our core temperature and processes taking place in the body.

Water can absorb a lot of heat and store it before it changes temperature. For this, our body uses water to help maintain our internal temperature, even with fever. In general, water tends to have a cooling effect because it thins and moves the blood which can carry heat to the surface of the body, the skin, for dispersal.

What is water? It's commonly defined as a colorless, transparent, odorless, tasteless liquid that is necessary for all life. Wow, doesn't sound too appetizing, does it? Regardless, if your water has a pronounced taste, it may bear investigating. The taste of water can change depending on its mineral content, which can cause a slight metallic taste. A low pH can also cause a metallic taste. Water normally has a pH of 7, which is considered a balance between alkaline and acidic, but it can vary from 6.5 to 8.5. Low pH water, called soft water, can result in a slight acidic taste. Contaminants in water may result in a slightly salty taste. Hard water tends to be high in minerals such as calcium.

While fire is a process, water is an element. To understand the element of water in Southern blood types, it is important to understand the nature of water, the importance of salt, and water's need for minerals. Water is the basis of all life and we can't live without it. About 60 percent of the human body is composed of water, and about three-quarters of the Earth's surface is water. Due to this fact, the element of water will have considerable influence on your health regardless of your dominant element. We all need water.

Water was central to early civilizations and is no less important today. Early man, depending upon hunting and gathering for survival, created settlements and villages close to creeks and rivers. This provided fish for food, drinking water for life, and fertile land for plants. Later as agriculture became an important factor in human civilization, flooding rivers left deposits of silt, which were necessary for the fertility of the land. Spring floods ensured a healthy fall harvest.

As populations increased, rivers and oceans also provided transportation and increased trade opportunities with neighbors. While ancient man built upon the water, Romans and Greeks learned to bring the water to them in the form of gravity-fed aqueducts and tunnels. This was a turning point in the movement and settlement of populations away from building along creeks, rivers, and the seas. Today, modern man has learned to control the waterways with a massive network of dams, canals, and reservoirs, ensuring a constant water supply to large inland cities and easily navigated, tamed rivers. The oceans, of course, are still wild.

Water plays a role in many religions around the world, as well as ancient mythologies. In the Christian religion, people who have been saved are baptized in water. Water washes away sin as the Great Flood washed away the sins of the world. In Hinduism, water has special spiritual cleansing powers, especially the water of the Ganges River. In some Native American tribes, all rivers and streams are held to be sacred and were never polluted or soiled. Too bad we don't acknowledge the importance and sacredness of water anymore; our water supply would be a lot less polluted.

In the mythologies of diverse cultures around the world, creeks, rivers, pools, ponds, lakes, and even the oceans were given personality traits that often described their natural cycles or areas of their stretch. Sometimes they were inhabited by magical creatures or spirits. There is the famous Lady of the Lake who gave the sword Excalibur to King Arthur and later, after his death, brought his body to Avalon. There are the Scottish Selkies and the Irish Roane, sea lions that could shed their skins and live with humans. There is the Loch Ness monster in Scotland; the water horse in Scandinavia; the Bunyip, evil spirits, in Aboriginal Australia; the water dragons in China; the Jengu, water spirits, of Cameroon; and the Uncegila, a water snake in Lakota mythology. The nymphs of ancient Greek mythology, along with the Sirens, lured sailors to their death. Throughout the world's cultures, there are water gods, water creatures, tales of warriors, stories of romances, and tales of the fountain of youth. Water itself could also have magical or healing properties. Achilles's mother tried to make him immortal by dipping him in the River Styx. It worked well except for the area on his heel where she held him. Ponce de Leon looked for the fountain of youth, but alas didn't find it.

Water soothes and heals. In Western civilization, the Greeks began the art of the public bath. While a basin might be used at home for personal cleanliness, the bath provided the opportunity for relaxation and submersion. The Romans elevated the public bath, providing large pools for bathing and relaxing, and showers for personal hygiene. These Greek and Roman baths were often built on or near hot mineral springs. Gender-segregated public baths can be found in Japan, Turkey, Russia, Hungary, and Italy. It was a way for people in the community to share relaxing, healing, and social time. Just a note: A commonality of public baths is that the participants are expected to remove dirt and grime by washing the body in a basin or showering before entering the baths for a soak.

Who doesn't love a good soak? Civilization has progressed to the point that almost anyone can have a private bath at home. Maybe with some Epsom salts or a drop of lavender essential oil? Soaking in water soothes the frazzled nerves and relaxes the tattered psyche. It's a return to the mother's womb, floating along without a care. It's a chance to release the tension in the shoulders and the tightness in the chest. A bath, either hot or cold, can also reduce pain and irritation in the muscles and help heal torn or injured muscles, ligaments, and tendons.

Water never goes away: It just moves somewhere else. Every drop of water that was ever on the Earth is still on the Earth. In the water cycle, large bodies of water such as oceans, rivers, and lakes are heated by the sun and the water evaporates into the sky. Here it condenses around dust particles, becoming liquid and forming clouds. When the air can't hold the condensation anymore, it falls to Earth as precipitation—rain, sleet, snow, hail. And then it starts all over again. Winds may blow the rain clouds here or there, making some areas rainier than others. Just remember that it takes water to make rain, which was another advantage of building towns close to water sources. Note also that water is the only element that can exist in all three states: liquid, gaseous, and solid.

Water always wins. It will wear away at the soil, rocks, and mountains, whether as a flash flood or a slow, patient drip. Over time, banks of creeks and streams are worn down, mountains are leveled, and boulders are shattered. Water deepens valleys and creates canyons. Both water and wind change the face of the Earth, but fire only temporarily changes the surface features. The same goes for water people, who have the ability to wear away at any situation until it's to their liking.

It is powerful. A tsunami displaces water with such force that the destruction can move past the shoreline to inland areas. Slow-moving thunderstorms cause flash floods that destroy homes, roads, and bridges and tear down trees. When water and wind unite, destruction can result. Wind pushes water to create waves across a lake; the faster the wind speed, the higher the wave. There are large waves and small ones, riptides, wild waves, and rogue waves. A hurricane, cyclone, or typhoon can cause high waves, high winds, storm surge, and tornadoes. Any of these storms are a force of nature that can take lives, wreak havoc on structures, and demolish forests. This might be a thought for the water/air personal relationship—sometimes there's going to be waves.

The gravitational pull of the moon and the sun creates tides on the ocean, with the moon having the greatest effect. These reliable waves rise and fall on shorelines around the world. Understanding the movement of the tides, incoming and outgoing, has always been important for sea travel. Flood tides are incoming to the shore and create high tides; ebb tides are outgoing and create low tides. A good ship's captain times leaving the harbor so that there is enough water to lift the ship, enough tide to move the ship, but not too much tide to decrease maneuverability. That takes some practice! This is a tip to water folks: Wait for the right flow before making major decisions that will affect your relationships.

Water is a power that can be harnessed. Dam a river and the water will drive a turbine and generator, creating hydroelectric powers. Run water over a water wheel and corn is ground in the grist mill. In this instance, water from a stream was often dammed to create a channel of water that flowed over the wheel. Abandoned mill ponds were great swimming holes in my youth.

Water is so vital that the human body can only live about three to five days before dehydration can result in death. We lose water through breath and sweat, in vomit and tears, and in urine and feces. The most common cause of death due to dehydration is diarrhea, especially in children and the elderly. Diabetes is the chronic illness most associated with dehydration. People in higher altitudes are also at a greater risk for dehydration due to the fact that we lose twice as much fluid through sweating and breathing here than at sea level. Signs of mild dehydration include dry mouth, lethargy, headache, dizziness, lack of tears, scant urine, and muscle weakness. Signs of serious dehydration include dry skin, low blood pressure, heart palpitations or straining heart, low blood pressure, dry skin, and fever. Get some water fast!

Hot, dry air and cold, dry air will cause loss of water. Heat also causes fluid loss. We must replace the water we lose to keep our organs and our bodies working efficiently. A good rule of thumb is to drink enough water to equal half your body weight in ounces each day. If you weigh 150 pounds, drink seventy-five ounces, and if you weigh 250 pounds, drink 125 ounces. Add another ten ounces for every six ounces of caffeine or alcohol you consume. This is extremely important to water folks.

On the other hand, too much water is poisonous. This is known as water intoxication, a dangerous situation and can be fatal. Drinking a large amount of water in a short period of time can result in a swift drop in sodium. Symptoms of water intoxication include confusion, disorientation, nausea, and vomiting, and changes in a person's mental state. In this situation, most people vomit up water as an immediate attempt by the body to slow down sodium loss. The rate at which the sodium falls is an important factor in the progress of symptoms through confusion, drowsiness, and then coma.

Water is one of our most polluted natural resources. It's estimated that in developing countries, 70 percent of untreated industrial wastes and sewage are dumped or discharged into waters, polluting the useable water supply, whether rivers, lakes, or coastal areas. Water is the universal solvent and is capable of dissolving more chemicals than any other liquid on Earth. Wherever water goes, so do chemicals, minerals, or nutrients. This is true in our bodies as well as on the land.

Contamination of our drinking water supplies is a serious health issue. Every time you turn on your tap, traces of birth control pills, high blood pressure medications, nitrates and other farm runoff, pesticides, and herbicides come spilling out your faucet. It's a water treatment plant, not a water purification plant. Municipal water treatment plants are charged with filtering out sediment and bacteria, removing excess minerals and contaminates, and sending the water to your household. If you have any doubts of this, just keep in mind the water fiasco in Flint, Michigan, which is still ongoing at the time of this writing. The improperly treated city water supply corroded old iron pipes with lead solder, which contaminated the city's drinking water with high levels of lead and iron. This effectively poisoned many of the citizens of Flint, especially vulnerable children.

Types of Water in the Body

In Southern Folk Medicine, water has a very broad meaning. Yes, it does mean that odorless, tasteless liquid that we can't live without, but that's not the only type of water in our bodies. According to folk tradition, the water element governs or influences most all fluids in the body. This includes mucus, extracellular fluid, urine, sweat, tears, amniotic fluid, saliva, pus, vaginal secretions, plasma, and semen. These are just a few types of water that make up 60 to 70 percent of our body. If all the water suddenly evaporated from our bodies, not too much substance would be left.

Unlike other nutrients, water is already broken down into its smallest components, which makes for quick and efficient absorption. Water molecules are so small that they are directly absorbed through the lining of the membranes. When you drink a glass of water, some water is absorbed from the mouth and stomach, but the majority is absorbed in the small intestines and enters directly into the bloodstream. About 10 percent of the water we drink makes it to the large intestine to aid in the elimination of wastes.

Blood and Lymph

Most of our blood and lymph is actually composed of water. In addition to carrying water to the cells, blood also carries proteins, sugars, fats, oxygen, and immune factors. Blood is our life stream. Importantly, the water that is absorbed in the small intestine to the blood stream flows through the arteries, arterioles, and then into capillaries that surround all cells. Once the blood reaches the capillaries, plasma, the watery portion of the blood, seeps into the space surrounding the cells and is now known as tissue fluid. Tissue fluid is composed of water and any molecules small enough to diffuse out of the tiny capillaries, such as proteins or glucose. Cells absorb water by osmosis, depending on how much sodium is present. Osmosis is the movement of water from an area of higher water concentration to one of lower concentration, which equalizes concentrations on either side of the membrane. Lymph also delivers fats to the cells.

After delivering water and nutrients to the cells, the tissue fluid and lymph will pick up cellular wastes and toxins and send them to the liver and kidneys for processing. Any water-soluble contaminants will make their way to the kidneys, which clean and filter the blood, and the waste is released as urine.

Lymph is a clear fluid that travels the body in the lymphatic system, which is just as complex as the circulatory system. If you've ever had a sunburn, lymph is the clear liquid in a water blister. It's also the oozing liquid you see when you've got a carpet burn or you've scraped your skin just enough for the lymph to be seen, but not deep enough to bleed. As mentioned earlier, lymph carries fats and nutrients to the cells and removes cellular wastes. Once the lymph leaves the cell, it heads back toward the heart, pausing along the way at lymph nodes, which filter the lymph fluid and remove foreign cells and debris. The lymph nodes also contain white blood cells, which address any bacteria in the fluid. The filtered lymph is slowly pushed toward the heart and eventually enters the thoracic duct and then the circulatory system.

There is no lymph pump, unlike the blood, which has the heart for a pump. Lymph fluid moves by muscle movement and deep breathing. To move your lymph, you must move, walk, exercise, rebound, or practice deep breathing. Dehydration can cause sluggish lymph movement. Certain types of massage can also move the lymph. Be conscious of this very important component of the body. Too little research is available on this amazing system as it has been totally ignored in favor of the circulatory system by conventional medicine. But not in traditional herbalism, which has a whole category of herbs known as lymphatics—cleavers, chickweed, red root, mullein, violet, prickly ash, and red clover are a few examples. Natural approaches to health have traditionally appreciated this otherwise undervalued system.

Urine

Urine is formed as blood is filtered through the kidneys to eliminate waste, maintain hydration, and ensure blood pH. At any given moment, about 20 percent of our blood is flowing through the kidneys. Not all the water that flows through the kidneys is released as urine. Some water, nutrients, and minerals are reabsorbed into the bloodstream in the capillaries surrounding the tubules. In a healthy person, all the glucose is reabsorbed; in a diabetic, sugar spills into the urine. In the final stage of urine formation, some minerals and ammonia are secreted, as are some medications and hormones.

The color of your urine may offer some clues to general health and hydration status. In general, pee should be slightly straw-colored to a bit yellow, but still transparent. If your urine is totally clear, you may be drinking too much water or not absorbing what you are drinking. Too much water will flush minerals from the body. If you think absorption is the issue, try increasing salt intake or adding a squeeze of lemon or lime to your water.

If your urine is dark yellow, dehydration may be an issue. Always, always see your healthcare provider if there is blood in your urine, which may indicate a kidney or bladder infection or irritation. If your pee is always foamy, there may be too much protein in your diet, which can damage the kidneys over time.

Bottom line: We often take for granted how much water we need each day. Find the amount of water that keeps your body hydrated without loss of minerals.

Mucus or Phlegm

The slippery slime of mucus is made by mucous membrane tissues that line any organ that connects to or interacts with the outside world—sinuses, inside of the eyelid, esophagus, bronchial tubes, lungs, stomach, gallbladder, small intestines, large intestines, bladder, uterine mucosa, vaginal mucosa, and penile mucosa.

When these mucous membrane tissues are irritated, they produce mucus. If you've ever had a cold, the snotty liquid dripping from your nose is mucus.

Mucus is composed of water, antibodies, antiseptic substances, salts, and a protein called mucin. It provides lubrication and protection to the mucous membrane tissue it covers. Healthy mucus is clear, thin, and watery. Any thickening or discoloration of the mucus can point to a health issue. Everyone who has ever had a cold has observed their snot going through color changes—clear, thick and milky, yellow and thick, and then green and thick, and in the same progression back to normal.

According to the old healers, canker is a type of mucus that results from sores, lesions, and areas of disease in the body, especially the bowels, though this can happen anywhere. As the sore goes through stages of change and bacteria and dead cells build in the area, the mucus can harden into small gravel or a lump. Canker must be softened to be removed. As a visual, think about tonsil stones or gallstones. Both are aspects of hardened mucus with some bacteria, dead cells, and possibly some calcium thrown in.

Mucus, also called phlegm, can be produced wherever there are mucous membrane tissues. Canker can be produced wherever there are sores or lesions in the body, including the spinal column or brain, and may also be referred to as dry pus in those cases. Large amounts of mucus or canker constrict tissues and restrict blood and lymph flow into an area. This reduced flow creates a "cold spot" within the area, or tissues that need warming, stimulating herbs to correct. Without improved blood and lymph flow into the area, anti-infective herbs or even antibiotics will have reduced effectiveness.

Resolving the Hardening

When mucus, lymph, or tissue fluid thickens and doesn't move, problems happen. Due to restricted fluid flow, these areas are deprived of nutrients, while at the same time cellular wastes are not being removed and are building in the area. Issues like fluid-filled cysts, simple ovarian cysts, fluid-filled breast cysts, mucous balls in the lungs, or mucus in the gut may result. The lack of movement restricts blood and lymph flow, constricts tissues, increases inflammation, and creates lingering problems, including soft masses. Increasing blood flow to the area can improve the situation.

Warming and stimulating herbs to bring blood into an area include cayenne, ginger, cloves, pine, black pepper, prickly ash, and peppermint.

Traditional herbs to soften masses include black walnut, chickweed, red clover, plantain, mullein, echinacea, poke root, burdock, and yellow dock.

Traditional herbs to move hardened stones include gravel root, marshmallow, goldenseal, yellow dock, yucca, slippery elm, hollyhock, and hydrangea.

The Nature of Water: Seeking Relationship

Water cannot exist in a natural state without minerals. Water must be in a relationship with other elements in order to be healthy. This is one of the hallmarks of water people, who find their greatest physical and emotional health within healthy relationships, including relationships with themselves.

Pure water, also known as distilled water, is composed of two hydrogen atoms and one oxygen atom. But this is an unnatural state for water. Water cannot live alone: It needs minerals to be complete. Sea water obviously has more sodium than fresh water, but both contain an assortment of other minerals. Water is a fickle lover and easily picks up pollutants such as herbicides, pesticides, and various contaminants from factory effluent systems and farm runoff. This is also a caution for water people who can too easily pick unhealthy or needy partners.

Because distilled water contains no minerals, it is aggressive. It is seeking relationship. This means that distilled water is always striving, always working, to return to its natural mineral state. If distilled water runs through metal pipes, it will corrode the pipes, drawing minerals to create balance. This is also the reason that distilled water is the perfect solvent. Distilled water is so aggressive that it will absorb carbon dioxide from the air, creating an acidic solution in place of its normal alkaline one. Personally, I have a strong concern that drinking distilled water for long periods of time may result in mineral deficiencies that could create health issues.

Water cannot exist alone, and its perfect companion is salt. It is a fatal and attractive attraction. Think about your salt shaker on a humid day. How long before the salt has absorbed the moisture from the air? Salt is in the oceans, our tears, blood, and sweat. Of course, our blood and tears don't have the same salinity as the ocean, which is much greater, which is why salt water can still sting the eyes.

Water follows salt anywhere—into the digestive tract, our tears, saliva, mucus, and blood plasma. Water follows salt into the very cell itself. Without salt, all the tissues in the body would lose their water. Dehydration and eventual death would occur. Without water, we will die. Without salt, we cannot utilize water. So, without salt, we will die. How much salt is too much? Medical science continues to argue on this point, but we all need some salt, and water folk are more sensitive than others. I caution wise use of salt for the water person, especially in regards to blood pressure.

Salt is an element of the Earth and in ancient days was most commonly derived from seawater. For our ancient ancestors, salt was scarce, hard to find, and worth its weight in gold. The word *salary* is actually derived from salt, so scarce it was considered a currency of commerce.

Native Americans dug salt from the Earth and would also burn various tree and plant roots to produce ash, which was used for salt. The most common plants used in this manner were hickory nut shells, wild grapevine, and gravel root. Solomon's seal root was also ground and added to food for salt. Te-lah-nay, a member of the Yuchi Indian tribe of Alabama, was taken to Oklahoma on the Trail of Tears. Homesick, she walked the long way home from Oklahoma back to Alabama over a five-year period. According to her descendent Tom Hendrix, when asked what she missed the most on her long journey home, Te-lah-nay answered, "Salt." Only modern man has unlimited access to limitless amounts of salt.

Salt is composed of the elements sodium (Na) and chloride (Cl), but depending on its source other minerals may also be present. Sodium is very active and attaches itself strongly and quickly to other elements. For this reason, sodium is not found in pure form in nature, but can be created in a laboratory setting with the aid of an electrical current. The most common form of sodium found in nature is soda or sodium carbonate. The most common form of sodium found in the human body is sodium chloride.

Sodium, like water, cannot exist alone in a pure form. That makes for a unique circumstance for relationship; neither can exist alone. Both need a relationship with something outside themselves to be whole. There is a caution here for water folk also.

Sodium carries an electrical charge, and for this reason it's known as an electrolyte. It's important for muscle contraction, including that of the heart, for nerve transmission, is used in the transportation of amino acids from the gut to the blood, and is needed to maintain normal water balance in the body, within and without the cells. We store extra salt in the bones as reserves for a rainy day. Sodium also reacts with the hydrogen in water, producing heat, which is the reason salt melts ice.

Sodium resides outside the cell membrane and potassium resides within the cell. The exchange of sodium and potassium—sodium moves inside the cell while potassium moves to the outside—creates an electrical charge that causes a nerve impulse or muscle contraction. A deficiency of sodium or potassium can affect muscles and nerves rapidly. Moving sodium from inside the cell to the outside of the cellular membrane also helps remove acid from the body.

Salt itself has many uses, including as a digestive aid. Have you ever been really nauseated and only something salty like a chip or cracker would satisfy you? The sodium chloride increases production of stomach acid, which can have a soothing effect when acid is low. Salt also attracts moisture, and salty foods can help you stay hydrated during times of illness or during pregnancy.

It is soothing to mucous membrane tissues and makes an excellent wash for wounds and the eyes. It creates an inhospitable environment for bacteria by drawing the water from their cell walls, which reduces their capacity for reproduction. Salt is also irritating to the tissues and is not suggested as a disinfectant except in emergency situations. Think about the saying "rubbing salt in their wounds," a common practice after the lashing of prisoners and slaves. This was a painful and inhuman experience, but rubbing the wounds with salt did have the effect of reducing risk of infection and may have saved lives, though it must have stung like crazy and caused massive scarring.

Salt inhibits the growth of yeast and allows the fermentation process to progress. For this reason, salt is used to make vegetable fermentations such as sauerkraut. Luckily, probiotic strains of *Lactobacilli,* what we call good bacteria, are resistant to salt and actually thrive in the salty environment if excessive salt isn't used. Using salt in vegetable fermentations also adds a bit of crunch to the finished product.

Too much salt is drying. It sucks the water right out of the tissues, which makes it an excellent food preservative. This drying effect can extend to our internal tissues as well, creating dry mucous membranes subject to erosions, abrasions, and ulcers. It has been theorized that the high rates of stomach cancer in Eastern Asia, particularly Korea, Japan, and China, are influenced by the amounts of salty foods consumed such as soy sauce, salty fish, and pickles.

Water is wet and salt is drying. They need each other to achieve stability and to reduce the aggression of each.

The Tastes of Salts

The taste of salt generally doesn't change facial expression like bitter does, but may have you reaching for a glass of water. It can cause mucus on the back of the tongue and increased salivation. The taste of salt is dependent upon the composition of the minerals in the mixture. There is earth salt, pink salt, black salt, beige salt, and gray salt, depending on the source and mineral composition. Regardless of your salt origin preference, make sure that you are getting adequate iodine in your diet.

Do all mineral salts taste salty? In general, the answer is no. Halite, also called rock salt, tastes salty because it's composed of sodium chloride. Hanksite, composed of sodium potassium sulfate carbonate chloride, also has a salty taste. But mineral tastes can be as varied as plant tastes. In Southern Folk Medicine, only minerals with a salty taste are considered influential in the salty blood type.

Other minerals may taste sweet or bitter. Lead and borax are said to taste sweet. Epsom salts taste bitter. Calcium tastes bitter. A little potassium chloride tastes salty, but too much tastes bitter. Pyrite tastes a bit like sulfur, which is actually more of a stinky smell than a taste, which is bittersweet. Iron and iodine both taste metallic, which is more of a quality rather than a taste, which is actually a bit sour bitter.

By the way, I am a fan of iodized salt. During my youth, I saw the massive thyroid goiters that would hang on women's necks due to lack of iodine. I know there are issues with our current salt supplies, such as the amount of sugar and anti-caking agents put in table salt, but the incidence of hypothyroidism related to iodine deficiency has dropped tremendously. If you aren't willing to use iodized salt, please investigate adequate sources of the vital nutrient.

Think about the nature of water and its relationship with salt and minerals as we discuss the traits of water people. Water cannot exist alone; it must have a companion (minerals). In a pure state, water is aggressive. Water follows salt anywhere. Sodium does not exist in a pure state in nature but must combine with other elements, such as chloride. Salt is drying; water is wet. Together they make balance. So the question is: Does salt pull the moisture from tissues or does the water follow the salt out of the tissues? Quite a metaphor for water people and their quest for the perfect relationship.

Water Traits

The element water is associated with the humor or body fluid of water and the taste of salt. Water plays a role in the development of mucus (phlegm) and is therefore associated with the mucous membrane tissues of the digestive tract, bladder, gallbladder, lungs, sinuses, and reproductive systems. It is also associated with the blood, lymph, tissue fluid, urine, and other water-based fluids in the body. Water is associated with the breasts, reproductive organs, feet, toes, kidneys, and the shaping of the physique. The water element is known as salty blood type in the Southern blood types.

Water always wins. Whether moving slow or fast, water gets its way, and so do water people. Water erodes mountain, cuts channels in solid rock, creates canyons, and causes massive destruction of man-made objects. Ultimately, nothing can withstand the power and tenacity of water, whether on the land or within relationships.

Water people prefer the path of least resistance, meaning the path in life with the fewest obstacles and most steady movement, but life doesn't always happen that way. For example, a creek will flow easily downhill fed by gravity until a resistance is introduced, like a landslide or big rock. The water will find a new path of flow around the obstacle or will wait and pool until there is enough water dammed behind the rock to begin to move it. That's water folks to a T.

To be in control of their lives, water people need good, strong boundaries; with those boundaries in place, they can manage any obstacles that might arise. Think about rivers, creeks, and streams. When water is within its banks, it makes its way to the sea, the ultimate destination of any moving water on this planet.

When water overflows it banks, there is diminished movement and momentum, and swampy, stagnant land results. It is the same with water people; you've got to keep moving to avoid stagnation.

Water people need strong boundaries defined by a belief system, a philosophy, or a set of rules to maintain their course in life. For some water folks, the beliefs and rules of institutions, religious or spiritual systems, social ethics, the military, or personal relationship rules will do this for them. They do well when connected to large groups of like-minded people. Think schools of fish, all swimming together with the same destination in mind, all turning at the same time, in the same way, and in the same direction.

When water people find their organization, their institution, church, or belief system, they truly *believe*. These are the people who have faith and belief and aren't always swayed by facts or figures. Their faith is strong, and things don't have to be proven to be believed. It's no accident that in the Age of Pisces (water), the symbol of Christianity is the fish. On the other hand, until they do believe, there is no stronger doubting Thomas than a water person.

Water people function well in institutions and organizations, such as the military, the church, corporations, or the law. These are all organizations where the rules and regulations are defined and everything is black or white. Water people have trouble seeing the gray areas of life, where things get muddy and boundaries blur.

The most dominant forces in the life of water people are their relationships. This could be their relationship to another person such as a friend, lover, or partner; their country; their church; their job; their family; or themselves. To water people, every human activity is about the inherent relationships within. Because water people understand relationships so well, they make excellent counselors, psychologists, investigative researchers, and detectives. They see and understand those hidden motives in relationships that may not be apparent to the other elements, especially fire and earth, who tend to take things at face value.

The primary hormones associated with water are reproductive hormones, oxytocin, serotonin, antidiuretic hormone, and aldosterone. Although these hormones may have either a cholesterol or protein base, their activity and end effect are relationship based. Water people often have a strong drive to reproduce, as do fire folk. But it's the relationships that result from this drive to produce, whether offspring or great works, that set folks upon their life course.

The primary neurotransmitter associated with water is oxytocin, which helps us bond with our mates in relationships and children when they are born. It's released by hugging or touching, during sex, childbirth, and breastfeeding. But, it's also the hormone that helps us bond with our herd, our group, our school of fish, with others like us. Oxytocin helps us relax, lowers blood pressure, and helps build trust with others. It increases empathy, and for this reason is often called the moral hormone.

Aldosterone helps maintain the salt and water balance in the body. It is made in the adrenal glands and released into the blood to signal the kidneys to reabsorb sodium back into the blood or sweat out excess sodium. Antidiuretic hormone helps the body hold onto or conserve water that would be lost through urine. Both are needed for healthy and balanced fluid movement and storage.

People with a dominant water element are emotional, intuitive, creative, and sentimental. They can often empathize and feel what another person is feeling. Water folks can also be a touch sympathetic, sometimes to the detriment of themselves or their own family, especially if a child is being neglected or harmed. It's quite easy for a water person to feel sorry for another. Because water folk are so empathetic and sympathetic, they often appear to be psychic, but they are just really picking up the cues and signals of how folks feel.

Water folks make excellent actors, writers, dancers, and artists, emoting or reflecting through their art. A water person becomes the role, becomes the part, becomes the character. This is a transformation and an amazing, believable one. In contrast, fire people, who also make good actors, dancers, and artists, project their same basic fire personality regardless of the character they are playing, and we love them for that.

When water people are in a trusted social group and feel safe, they are fun, friendly, witty, and social. In a new or unknown situation, water people tend to get a feel for things before speaking or interacting. They are so empathetic to others' feelings that they must protect themselves.

Water people often reflect those around them. Think about being on a boat on a lake and looking down at the water. What do you see? Only a reflection of yourself staring back. This reflective ability allows the water person to be in a large group and not stand out or get noticed. But it also creates a secretive side of water because as long as they are reflecting, you never truly know them.

Water people have amazingly sharp minds and a way of seeing and using logic in a manner that is very hard to argue against, especially for fire or air people. This is why they make good lawyers and judges, and politicians and preachers. Water people don't mind living alone, without personal relationship, if they have an institution such as church to connect with and if they have a strong relationship with themselves.

Water folks work well in groups and need the social interaction that work can bring. Corporations provide another strong working environment for water folk. They innately understand the logistics of working within the corporate environment—just a different type of relationship.

Water is generally cooling to the body, mind, and emotions. It lulls and soothes, softens and forms. After the initial passion of a new relationship has passed, water folks settle rather coolly into the relationship for the long haul. Like water needs minerals, water people need a relationship and will go to great lengths to keep a relationship even if it's an unhealthy one. Water people often cling to their relationships the way water clings to the skin—until they feel it's detrimental to their own health.

Water folks are medium boned with a medium build, similar to the build of fire. One main difference is muscle definition: Water folk generally don't have well-defined muscles, even after working out. This doesn't mean that they don't have strong muscles or body; they certainly do. The shape of the water muscle often appears smooth, without the cut that fire might see. In comparison, fire folk can have good muscle definition that shows each and every little indentation in the muscle body.

Fire and water make steam. Fire is the element that reduces water by evaporation, but this does not destroy water; rather it destroys the fire instead. Water just evaporates to become rain and return to Earth. Fire and water folk have to really work hard to have a healthy relationship, because over time, the water will reduce the fire; it's natural law. Air makes waves over the water and can speed up the evaporation process. Air and water folk often have a tumulus relationship but an interesting one. When the air is blowing, it adds extra energy to the movement of the water. Earth and water are another interesting combination. When earth is strong, like the bank of a creek, then water is supported and can flow and be productive. If water overflows the relationship boundaries, the creek bank, they make mud, resulting in stagnation and swampy land, and potentially a stagnant relationship. Water folk are often the happiest with other water folk who understand the beauty of relationship in all its many facets.

Like fire people, water people must move to be healthy. Physical activity moves the water and the lymph and helps avoid stagnation. Water people have the most energy when eating chicken and fish, beans, and watery fruits such as berries. Heavy starches and grains should be eaten in limited quantities due to lack of adequate digestive enzymes for these foods. The water person is sensitive to absorbing salt from food and may not need additional salt when cooking or at the table. They need to protect the kidneys and reproductive systems, and are prone to infections and cysts in both areas. They also tend to have a sweet tooth and should be cautious eating processed sugar, opting for honey or maple syrup instead. Processed sugar can also affect insulin release, blood sugar levels, and the kidneys.

Excess Water

Excess water shows in the personality as depression, self-pity, and emotional angst. The immediate outward show of emotion for excess water is crying. Tears will flow at any opportunity.

As the water builds, there is a tendency to become apathetic, cold, and unemotional. Here we have the expression "a cold fish." Excess water people must be cautious to avoid becoming emotional tsunamis that wash over everything and everyone in their paths. They must also be cautious to avoid self-medicating with alcohol or other drugs because addiction could be an issue. Excess water people may lose their intuitive feel and develop rigidity in an effort to bring the excess water back into control.

On a physical level, excess water presents as cold and damp, with not enough fire; air may also be low. A person might exhibit bladder or kidney problems, and irritations and infections of the mucous membrane tissues. Chronic obstructive pulmonary disorder (COPD), emphysema, colds, coughs, and sinus and lung congestion may also result from excess water. In the cardiovascular system, congestive heart failure, high blood pressure, heart valve problems, and stroke may be present. Other signs of excess water are ovarian cysts, swollen extremities, body cysts, and excess saliva or tears. The tongue may be pale but swollen.

Increasing fire using stimulating or heating herbs and mild diuretics to dry the excess water can be very helpful. Stimulating herbs include ginger, cayenne, prickly ash, smartweed, lobelia, and mints.

Drying herbs include sage, sumac, bayberry, gravel root, juniper berry, Queen Anne's lace, and cleavers.

Deficient Water

As I mentioned earlier, when an element is under stress, the person may show the traits of their opposite element. Deficient water can present with elements of fire and vice versa. In general, because the opposite element isn't the true personality of the person, staying in the opposite, fire, will only create further deficiency. It's handy to review the opposite element when investigating ongoing patterns of dysfunction or personality changes.

On a personality level, a water person with deficient water element may be easily irritated, show temper, and be impatient and angry. They are often curt and generally like to boss other people around, especially their family and friends. They may also scream and yell and say very hurtful things to those they love. Deficient water can become controlling and overly critical.

Deficient water people know how to go for the emotional jugular and will hold nothing back in their emotional attacks if they feel threatened or attacked themselves. In this scenario, they don't play fair. They may also display jealousy, especially if any of their relationships appear to be threatened.

Deficient water may present physically as thin, dry, and weak hair, skin, and nails. In extreme cases the skin may be wrinkled and leathery as the water is lost to fire or air. Think of the stereotype of the salty dog, the old mariner of New England. The blood may lack moisture, creating thick blood, which can lead to blood clots, stroke, cardiovascular disease, and heart attack.

Moistening herbs and foods will help bring deficient water back into balance. Moistening herbs include slippery elm, marshmallow, hollyhock, chickweed, plantain, oats, aloe vera, and American ginseng.

❧ ELEVEN ❧

Air or Wind: Sour Blood

A nation that destroys its soils destroys itself. Forests are the lungs of our land, purifying the air and giving fresh strength to our people.

—Franklin D. Roosevelt

DADDY WAS A WHISTLER. He whistled whole songs in complex multirhythms that fell melodious on the ears. Daddy whistled when he was happy; he whistled when he was sad; and he whistled just to pass the time of day. He whistled to call the dogs, to get the attention of us kids, and to praise something beautiful. He whistled to imitate birds. Daddy had a whistle for almost any situation or occasion. He whistled down the street when shopping, and passersby would comment on what a fine whistler he was. He whistled instead of applauding at a ballgame or school event. I remember in second-grade recital, I was dressed as a tulip along with two other girls, and we sang a song about Holland. When we finished our song, I could hear Daddy's whistle over the applause and I was mighty pleased. Importantly, Daddy would whistle when he was nervous or upset. In those days, whistling was considered a manly musical art, and very few women whistled in public. Try as I may, I could never whistle at all. It is now a lost art.

He also played the harmonica when the mood struck. Daddy could make that harmonica cry and wail; he could make it sound like a choo-choo train; and he could make it sing the blues. He could also make the harmonica sound so sweet that you almost wanted to cry. It's safe to say that Daddy had a musical bent.

Along with his brothers, Daddy had a reputation as a ballplayer, both basketball and baseball. If it was round and moved through the air, Daddy could control it. He was a natural pitcher and natural switch-hitter, and many are the stories that have been told about his expertise. Daddy played some type of ball in local leagues until his mid-fifties. He probably would have kept on playing, but bursitis in his shoulder slowed him down. I watched him pitch a game with his glove under his arm. It was amazing how fast he could put on that glove once the ball left his hand.

Daddy made a living as a carpenter. He was a good framer and joiner, did fairly well on remodels, and managed to stay as busy as the local economy would allow. Due to the hard work and heavy hammering, Daddy had freakishly large forearms and very thick and calloused hands. They were amazing. His skin was bronze from the sun and his hair was so black that it had blue highlights. In his youth, Daddy was a good-looking man.

In addition, Daddy was also the local handyman. If someone's stove stopped working, they called Daddy. If someone needed an element replaced in a hot water heater, they called Daddy. If someone had a leaking roof, they called Daddy. If someone's iron stopped working, they called Daddy. Sometimes, Daddy was so busy with other folks' repairs that our house suffered, much to Mama's disconcertment.

Daddy usually either whistled or sang as he milked the cow. We didn't own a barn or a pasture, but we did own a cow. Our neighbors, the Albrights, let us pasture our cow and use a stall in their barn for milking. Daddy milked mornings before he went to work and evenings when he got home. If you've ever owned a milk cow, you know how this can tie you to the land. A cow has to be milked or mastitis, infection, can set in.

Good raw milk, or sweet milk as we called it, is absolutely delicious. We almost always had a gallon in the refrigerator unless the cow was dry. A glass of raw whole milk is filling, nutritious, and counts as food, not a beverage. One of Daddy's favorite meals was a glass of cornbread and milk. In this classic Southern dish, cornbread is crumbled into a glass or bowl of milk. Sometimes, a bit of bacon or fried potatoes rounded out the meal. Raw milk is chock-full of enzymes and nutrients that are destroyed in the pasteurization process. Just thinking about the taste of a cold glass of raw milk almost—just almost—makes me wish I had a cow.

Daddy developed a cough and a pain in his ribs, and both grew worse over time and nothing he did seemed to improve his symptoms. After a visit to the doctor, Daddy was diagnosed with tuberculosis. This was the day that changed our family forever.

In those days, a tuberculosis diagnosis meant confinement at a TB sanitarium. Daddy was given one week to get his affairs in order, and the county sheriff came to escort him to the TB sanitarium in Gadsden. He tried to appear strong during this week, but he was a nervous wreck, and there was a tremendous amount of anxiety about his diagnosis. Tuberculosis was a weakness in the Light family.

With Daddy gone, it was a tough time for our family. In those days there were no social services, and no food stamps or other aid available. This is when Mama began cleaning houses because the cotton fields were gone and we needed the money. Our whole family had to be tested for tuberculosis and take isoniazid (INH) for six months as a preventative measure, with regular checks by the local health department to ensure compliance. I went to work at age fourteen to help support the family. As a matter of fact, each of us kids did whatever we needed to help our survival.

My sister tried milking the cow in Daddy's stead, but it was tough times. Mama sold the cow because we needed the cash more than we needed the milk. A week later, the person who bought the cow returned and wanted his money back. The cow had been tested and had tuberculosis. It had to be put down.

The huge question: Did we get tuberculosis from the cow? It wasn't ever tested when Daddy bought it from a neighbor; we simply started drinking the milk. Or did Daddy give the cow tuberculosis? It's more likely that the cow had tuberculosis and we had been drinking the infected milk for quite some time. To this day, I won't drink raw milk unless I know it has been tested for tuberculosis and other bacteria. The stakes are too high, and I've already been down that road.

In typical Air fashion, Daddy was high strung and nervous on the inside but tried not to show it on the outside. When the stress of a situation was more than he could bear, Daddy would let out a sigh, look the other way, and get up and leave the room. Flight was his natural way of dealing with stress, especially emotional stress. Don't get me wrong, Daddy could fight if need be, but that wasn't his natural urge. Maybe that came from being in the middle of seven boys. You learned to keep the peace.

Daddy loved to read paperback Western novels and loved Zane Grey. He liked watching Westerns and Army movies on television. Daddy would watch science fiction movies, especially if there was action and adventure to be had. One of my best memories is falling asleep on the couch on Saturday nights to the sound of the blazing guns of a war movie or cowboy shootout. Me on the couch and Daddy in his easy chair. It was special times.

Daddy taught me about the woods and to love books. We hunted ginseng and other herbs, and on these walks I learned about the wild plants. Other times, we just ambled along in the woods not looking for anything special, just enjoying nature. The woods quieted his airy soul, grounded him, and let him leave worries behind, at least for awhile. Books allowed him to escape into other times and places. Both aspects, I truly understand and love.

Daddy didn't come home from the TB hospital but found a new love instead—his affection blew in a different direction. This broke Mama's heart and wreaked havoc on our family in more ways than can be explained. After being gone for ten years, and all us kids grown and gone from home, Daddy came knocking on Mama's door and she gladly opened it. Daddy tried to pick up where he'd left off and in some ways he did. In other ways, things were never going to be the same. The blowing winds of his emotions and attention settled into a nice gentle breeze directed at Mama and they were as happy as air and water can be until his death.

Daddy became an amazing grandfather, much loved and beloved by all his grandchildren. He taught them gardening and how to grow giant tomatoes, how to hammer a nail into a piece of wood, how to watch out for snakes, how to walk in the woods, how to hit a ball, and how to shoot a hoop. He was affectionate, loving, and supporting. All the qualities of a good father and grandfather. I miss our time together terribly. This one is for you, Daddy.

Air or Wind

In Southern Folk Medicine, there is air and there is wind. Sometimes the two terms are used interchangeably, but here I'd like to make a distinction. Air has no form and is invisible. It takes up space, can fill a container, and exert pressure. It can suspend other particles within itself. We can't live without air, as it contains the gases required for human life.

Wind is moving air, which is also invisible in and of itself, but you can see the effects of its passage and you can sometimes see the things it carries, like dust, smog, or garbage. This is an important concept in Southern Folk Medicine. Wind carries things; it moves things. Air isn't fire, but wind and air can carry fire's heat. Air isn't water, but wind and air can carry water vapor, and wind over lakes causes waves. Air isn't earth; wind and air can carry dust and dirt for miles. Air holds things and wind moves them. That's an important concept in Southern Folk Medicine—there is air, and then there is wind.

Air is traditionally defined as the gases needed for life. Wind is traditionally defined as the movement of those gases. We pass wind after eating beans. We "get wind of something" that's new information that we didn't have before. A person who is three sheets to the wind is drunk on their butt. You can stand straight in the wind and risk snapping or you can bend with the wind, which is somewhat like going with the flow, but not exactly. Once the wind has passed you can straighten, but you never know where the flow of water will take you. A job, task, or relationship that's going nowhere is like pissing in the wind or spitting in the wind, take your choice of fluids. A second wind is when you're already tired but get another burst of energy close to the finish line. Running hard until you are gasping for breath is called being winded. Anyone who is "like the wind" is sure to break your heart because they come and go, physically and emotionally, and you never seem to know what's going on in the relationship. Throwing caution to the wind is taking a big risk or chance.

In traditional Southern Folk Medicine, any movement within the body falls under the domain of air. Eating too many beans gives you wind, which is the crampy pain felt as the gases work their way through the colon. Their expulsion is known as passing gas, which often has an odor similar to swamp gases, slightly sulfurous. This is the type of pain that comes and goes, just like the wind.

In addition to the gut, you can have wind in any joint, especially the fingers, in the leg muscles, shoulders, neck, eyes, and head. Any pain that comes and goes can be described as wind. Any unseen movement in the body is also under the domain of air. This is especially true of the nerves. Back then, no one knew exactly how the nerves worked, but knew they were there. I don't know how many times Mama would say, "You're getting on my last nerve." Or someone would have a "nervous breakdown" or say, "My nerves are shot."

Wind, often working with fire, moves the body. From the creation of energy in the Krebs cycle to the movement of the fluids in our body, wind contributes. Without oxygen in cellular respiration, there would be no production of ATP energy. Here's a perfect example of air and fire working together in the body. What a team!

This view of air and wind definitely has its origins in the humoral system, but there is another influence on the concept of wind in Southern Folk Medicine, and that is the Native American influence. Here, I can only speak of generalities because each tribe had different legends and beliefs, especially about the wind.

Like other parts of nature, wind was considered a force unto itself and separate from the air. If you've ever seen a tornado, you certainly can believe this to be true. In the ancient Creek tribes, some people were masters of the wind who would bring storms and tornadoes against the enemy in battle. The wind could bring the words and signs of the Creator to the tribe, and special people within the tribe could hear and communicate with this wind language. The four directions were based on the four winds and considered a symbol of power and life. The wind could bring illness, especially to someone who had committed a transgression within the tribe. The wind could follow you, the way smoke from a campfire does, for good or ill. Winds can be angry or gentle depending upon the mood of the Creator.

According to Creek legend, the wind can take human form and did so to have children. The Iron Monster stole his children and took them across a great river, where they were killed and cast into the waters. Finally, the wind found his dead children and fought with the Iron Monster, but couldn't kill him by normal means. So Wind blew a special smoke on Iron Monster and killed him in this manner. Unfortunately, when Wind brought his children back to life, they had been changed. Instead of leaving them, Wind stayed with them, promising, at some point, to rise and sweep across the Earth, destroying all in his path to avenge what had been done to his children.

In some Native American mythology, the plant most associated with the wind was tobacco. Smoking a pipe for pleasure was common in many Southeastern tribes among men, women, and children, as well as smoking a pipe for ceremony. Legends about the wind often include blowing smoke from a pipe to subdue or kill enemies. Here's another example of fire and air working together: You can't light a pipe and blow smoke without a little fire.

In West Africa, the wind can carry supernatural forces or invisible humans that attack people and can cause physical illness and mental health issues. This is called a bad wind or foul wind.

The Air We Breathe

Air and wind have no form but can carry heat or cold. Heat causes the molecules in the air to move faster and faster; cold causes them to move slower and slower. Air also reacts to atmospheric pressure. The closer to sea level, the warmer the air. The higher the elevation, the colder the air.

What is air? Air is that invisible, formless mixture of gases that sustains our life on Earth. We can live without water for several days, but we can only live without air for a few minutes. Air is what makes our world, the Earth, inhabitable to human life, and the lack of it makes other worlds uninhabitable. Try living on Mars or the Moon without oxygen or the gravity to hold the atmosphere in place and see what happens.

The air we breathe is a mixture of nitrogen, oxygen, carbon dioxide, water vapor, and other trace gases. Trace gases, such as argon, krypton, helium, neon, radon, and xenon, make up less than 1 percent of the remaining mixture. All the gases in the atmosphere get mixed by the wind and cover the Earth in a five- to six-mile-deep layer. Other substances in the air include pollens, dust, smoke, salt particles, chemicals, spores, bacteria, and viruses, all of which can affect our ability to breathe and our health. Air people should be cautious about any impediment to breathing. They are prone to seasonal allergies, food sensitivities, and feel the ill effects of odors and perfumes. Fresh air is one of the best medicines for air people.

The three most important gases needed for survival are oxygen, nitrogen, and carbon dioxide. We breathe in oxygen that combines with nutrients in our cells and releases ATP energy. While we can breathe pure oxygen for short periods of time, too much pure oxygen is poisonous. We breathe in air, use the oxygen in it, and release carbon dioxide and water vapor as waste products in respiration.

Plants are our partners in breathing, especially trees. In the photosynthesis process, plants breath carbon dioxide and with water create food and energy. They release oxygen and water vapor back into the atmosphere. About half the oxygen on the planet is produced by trees and land plants, and the other half is produced by phytoplankton, or algae, in the oceans. One tree produces enough oxygen for ten people to breathe. To top that off, trees also breathe in polluted air and breathe out clean air, the best air purification on the planet. How this happens is a mystery, but a wonderful one. Air people do well surrounded by plants, and benefit from both the exercise and fresh air of nature walks and gardening.

What happens to all that nitrogen we breathe? Since we can't use nitrogen from the air, we immediately exhale most of it. What's left circulates around our bodies along with the oxygen and is absorbed by the tissues. The heart, lungs, and abdominal tissues absorb nitrogen very fast, but stored fat, cartilage, and joints are slow to saturate. The amount of nitrogen saturation in the tissues is important to divers or people with impaired lung functioning.

Nitrogen is necessary to convert protein into amino acids, but we can't use nitrogen gas for this. Instead, we must use the nitrogen found in plants known as fixed nitrogen, and legumes are especially adapted for this purpose. Plants can take nitrogen from the air, and with the aid of bacteria, fix it at their roots, which also improves the fertility of the soil.

Every cell in our body requires oxygen to produce ATP energy in the oxidative process discussed in the chapter on fire. Oxygen helps fund the processes that contract our muscles during work or exercise. If the muscle doesn't have enough oxygen, then lactic acid is produced instead of energy. After physical activity, oxygen helps restore energy reserves and clears out lactic acid buildup.

Oxygen helps repair our cells by providing additional energy sources for wound repair or cell turnover. Not enough oxygen and the wound won't heal; too much oxygen and the wound won't heal. Like everything else in our bodies, it's all about the balance. Oxygen is also needed for the formation of new tissue. It is used by the liver in the detoxification process and metabolism of toxins and drugs. The liver actually requires more oxygen than any other organ, followed by the brain and then the heart.

The best way to get more oxygen into your body is to breathe properly. Breathing consists of two phases, inspiration and expiration. For inspiration, take a deep breath while expanding the diaphragm and lower rib cage outward, which increases the volume of the lungs while lowering the air pressure. It's easier to breathe outdoors where the air pressure is greater. Indoors, the air pressure is lower and sometimes, in well-insulated houses or shopping malls, we can't wait to get outside and take a deep breath of fresh air.

For expiration, let out the air while relaxing the diaphragm and intercostal muscles. This decreases the volume of the lungs and increases air pressure inside the lungs, forcing out the air. As the diaphragm relaxes, the chest cavity gets smaller; intercostal muscles squeeze the rib cage, which causes the lungs to begin collapsing as the air is pushed up and out of the body.

The influence of the air element on the lungs and respiratory tract is a given in physiology as well as traditional folk medicines. Air people are often very sensitive to air pollution, moldy houses, odors and scents, and cleaning chemicals, and should never smoke cigarettes.

Air folk use their sense of smell to warn of potentially damaging chemicals or bad air. These folks also unconsciously will smell or sniff their food before eating. This is especially true of air children, who will smell their food before taking a bite. Because they are so sensitive, air children do best with home-cooked meals. Fast food tends to smell bad to them. If it's in the air, then they are aware of it.

The Wind That Blows: All About the Nervous System

Air also influences the brain and the nervous system. At first glance, there may not seem to be a connection, but let's look a bit deeper. The brain is the control center of the central nervous system, which also includes the spinal cord and a gigantic network of nerves that wind through the body. It's the source of the wind.

For the brain to function at peak performance, it needs a constant supply of two substances: glucose and oxygen. With low oxygen levels, the brain may have trouble determining where to send blood to muscles and tissues.

About 70 percent of the brain is composed of water. Of the remaining 30 percent dry matter, about 60 percent of that is composed of lipids or fats, including cholesterol, essential fatty acids, vitamins A, D, and E, and phospholipids. While the brain's structure is dependent upon lipids, it must have a steady supply of glucose and oxygen for activity. Have you ever wondered why you get so hungry when you are working hard, studying, or learning something new? Your brain is in overdrive and requires fuel for thought. That's why it's easy to reach for the carbohydrates in these situations.

The brain uses about 25 percent of the oxygen we breathe in. That's quite a percentage considering its mass in comparison to, say, the liver or the large muscles in the legs. Lack of oxygen to the brain is called brain hypoxia and can be caused by smoke inhalation, choking, cardiac arrest, carbon monoxide poisoning, drowning, stroke, and any other condition that restricts oxygen flow to the brain. Mild symptoms include those that are often called brain fog—poor judgment and poor decision making, inability to think, and clumsiness or lack of coordination. Severe symptoms lead to death. Ways to increase oxygen to the brain include exercise, meditation, deep breathing, drinking adequate water, and antioxidants from food.

Without the central nervous system and the brain, your senses won't function. Hearing, seeing, smelling, tasting, and touching would not exist. Neither would dreaming, breathing, laughing, running, sleeping, jumping, singing, remembering, painting, writing, or spitting. And neither would pain, pleasure, fear, hope, love, despair, depression, happiness, or any emotions. There would be no thought and no action.

Wind is the movement of information along the neural pathway. It can manifest in the personality as any emotion or physically as pain and discomfort. Wind is in charge of fight-or-flight and the stress reaction. It's all about the nervous system and how information moves around the body. Air carries information and wind moves the information.

Nerves are thin threads of cells, or neurons, that run throughout the body. They carry messages back and forth just the way telephone wires and computer lines do. There are three types of nerves: sensory, motor, and interneurons. Sensory nerves send messages to the brain and central nervous system, and are linked to the sense of touch and feeling. Motor nerves carry messages back from the brain to all the muscles and glands in your body, which tell the muscles and glands what to do and when to do it. For example, when you touch a hot surface, sensory nerves let the brain know that the surface is hot to touch. The motor nerves carry the signal back to the hand to move away from the hot surface. All this happens in an instant. Interneurons are found only in the central nervous system and connect neuron to neuron.

All along the length of a nerve are synapses, the junctions between two nerve cells. Synapses are separated by a space called the synaptic cleft, which is just an open space (air) or narrow gap along the nerve. When a nerve impulse moves along a nerve, the impulse has to jump the open space or cleft to continue along its route. Neurotransmitters are released across the synaptic cleft to carry the nerve message across the gap. Think of neurotransmitters like helicopters that are lifting the message from one side of the open space to the other. The neurotransmitters can inhibit or stimulate the next neuron, depending on the message being sent.

Neurotransmitters that cross the cleft or gap bind with receptor sites, which ensures the transmission of the message along the nerve. They are only active a short time before being inactivated and reabsorbed (reuptake). About forty-one known neurotransmitters have been identified, but the most well-known are acetylcholine, noradrenaline, dopamine, histamine, glycine, oxytocin, gamma-aminobutyric acid (GABA), and serotonin. Some neurotransmitters are excitatory and stimulating, and others are inhibitory and relaxing. The dominant air person should be cautious with too much stimulation, which can release excitatory hormones in excess and the feeling can become addicting. Think adrenaline junkies.

Diseases and disorders of the nervous systems are generally considered air or wind disorders, including Parkinson's disease, ALS, neuromuscular disorders, and palsy. For example, Parkinson's disease is due to a deficiency in the neurotransmitter dopamine, and the signal can't cross the air space or gap. The majority of the neurotransmitters are made from protein. Without neurotransmitters, the chemical messengers of the nervous system, information from one brain cell to another or one neuron to another won't be sent or received. Mood and mental health disorders are also considered air or wind disorders. Sometimes these are due to neurotransmitter issues, and sometimes they are due to trauma, nutritional deficiencies, or injury.

Dominant-air people are prone to anxiety in social situations and performance anxiety while in school or at work. As air folk master their chosen area of study or profession, the anxiety is greatly reduced and replaced by expert knowledge and skills. Still, the self-esteem of an air person is often bound in what they know. Knowledge is an important asset to air folk.

Our Senses

The smell of baking bread; the memory of an exceptional moment; or the soft touch of a baby's skin. These experiences are possible because of one organ—the brain. Take a moment to experience your own senses. Close your eyes. What do you hear? Keep your eyes closed and concentrate on your fingertips. What do you feel? Take a deep breath. What do you smell? Now open your eyes. What do you see? Pour yourself a glass of juice or make a cup of herbal tea. What do you taste?

In today's modern world, our senses are constantly being bombarded with auditory and visual signals. How does our brain pick and choose what is important and what is trivial? Sometimes it can't or has trouble doing so, and problems result.

Our senses are classified into two categories: general senses and special senses. Receptors that are spread throughout the body, such as in the skin, give rise to general senses. Specialized receptors limited to certain sites give rise to special senses. General senses monitor touch, pressure, temperature, and pain. Other general receptors provide information about the position of the body and the length and tension of skeletal muscles.

The special senses include smell, taste, hearing, equilibrium, and sight. Each of the special senses correlates with specific structures in the body, for example, taste with taste buds or hearing and equilibrium with the ears. Each sense also has a particular mechanism for action and multiple aspects to its function.

In air folk, the senses are acutely tuned for fight-or-flight, especially hearing and smell. Both these senses are carried on the wind. Sound would not exist without the molecules in the air to carry it, and therefore there is no sound in empty space. Smell is a different kettle of fish. Smell can travel through space on gaseous molecules that move by diffusion across the emptiness, making it not empty anymore. Gases and physical particles can exist in a vacuum but tend to dilute across the vastness. Astronauts have reported a distinct smell of cooking meat after a spacewalk, and, reportedly, the moon has its own smell. Interesting.

The Nature of Air

Air is associated with the humor or body fluid of blood, the color of red, and the taste of sour or acid. Moving air is called wind, and the two terms, air and wind, are often used interchangeably in Southern Folk Medicine, though have somewhat different meanings. Air governs the brain, nervous system, lymph, lungs, shoulders, kidneys, bladder, lower back, legs, ankles, and circulation. It is responsible for the movement of fluids, gases, and nerve impulses through the body. It is also responsible for thought and the movement of neurons and neurotransmitters. The air element is also known as sour blood in the Southern blood types.

To understand the nature of the air element, it is important to understand the taste of sour and the digestion of protein. It's also important to understand the nature of stress. Because air governs the nervous system, it influences how we react to stress and our neurotransmitter activity, and has an especially strong effect on the sympathetic nervous system, which governs fight or flight.

Let's start with how the body digests protein and the taste of sour. Protein cannot be absorbed in the complex state in which it appears in food. Once we take in a protein food, our body must break it down into its constituent amino acids for utilization. Unlike carbohydrate digestion, which begins in the mouth, protein digestion begins in the stomach. Therefore, to digest animal protein, adequate hydrochloric acid is required. If you have normal stomach acid, this isn't an issue. If stomach acid is low, then protein digestion is going to be impaired. Some people have naturally low stomach acid, but many folks have low stomach acid due to antacid prescription medications designed to soothe acid reflux. These medications impair protein digestion and synthesis, as well as mineral absorption.

Until fire became common, our ancestors ate their food raw, including animal protein. Raw meat is fibrous and tough, and just doesn't pack the nutritional punch our brains and bodies needed to evolve. Our early ancestors spent hours and hours pounding their food with rocks and then chewing and chewing in order to receive enough nutrition to survive. But luckily, someone, most likely a raw meat eater, discovered fire and decided to throw some food on it. Or, more likely, decided to eat the cooked carcass of an animal left behind after a natural brush fire.

Eating raw meat with its inherent fatty acids made our ancestors smarter and allowed them to expand their territory and migrate across the land. But eating cooked meat was even better. Cooking meat liberates energy, makes it softer and easier to digest, and releases the protein in muscle tissue. Fire also allowed meat to be cut into strips and dried for future use, so the whole animal didn't have to be consumed within a short span of a few days.

As humans ate more meat, the body developed muscle for hunting, the brain grew bigger, and the digestive tract grew smaller. A longer digestive tract is needed to digest grains and plant materials; a shorter one works fine for meat-eating. This is most obvious in the animal world. Herbivores have the longest digestive tract, omnivores a shorter one, and carnivores a very short one. Think cow, black bear, and tiger. Modern man definitely has a shorter digestive tract than these animals, not as short as a true carnivore but longer than a true herbivore. We are somewhere in the middle.

For ancient man, enhancing the digestion and assimilation of protein, whether from plant or animal sources, improved repair from injury, recovery from illness, and overall longevity. Protein comprises the building blocks of most of our cells, including organ tissue, blood cells, bones, skin, hair, immune system, and muscle. We tend to use protein as we take it in. If we don't need the protein, then it's not broken down into amino acids, but rather, the calories are sent to storage as fat. The only storage site for protein is muscle, and that storage form is limited. This is why you lose muscle mass during an illness such as the flu. If you're sick and can't eat, then the body will cannibalize muscle tissue as a source of the vital amino acids needed for healing.

In addition to repair and rebuilding activities, protein is also used to manufacture enzymes, the sparks of life. Enzymes help break down our food, gobble up bacteria, and function as catalysts in many metabolic processes. They are also required to modulate the production of energy by mitochondria. Enzymes are only catalysts; they are not changed nor consumed in any reactions. They are so specific that only one enzyme can perform one specific function. There are no generalized enzymes; therefore, we need lots and lots of them. And this means that we need a sustained protein source to fund their manufacture.

Air people have a high requirement for good-quality protein whether from animal or plant sources, and it's important that it's available in the diet. They also do well with beans, whole grains, eggs, and fresh vegetables. Dairy may not be readily digested, and so its addition to daily protein may be limited.

The Taste of Sour

When we eat something sour, it makes our mouth pucker and we immediately start salivating. Our tongue will curl to funnel the spit-laden sourness from our mouths. Our lips pucker and we cringe. The reaction protects us from spoiled or unripe foods, and the taste is enhanced in certain fruit acids and fermented foods.

Food preparation techniques involving sour marinades partially evolved to help render tough animal tissue more tender, moist, and easily digested, plus they add flavor and mask the strong taste of wild game and aged meat. Marinades typically contain something sour, such as vinegar, sour milk, fruit juices, herbs, or wine, to help soften the tissue and bring moisture. Because marinades penetrate slowly, they may take several hours to be effective, and then the outside of the meat may be more sour and tender than the inside.

Another traditional foodway to help digest protein is to cook meat with fruits and herbs to increase tenderness. Think about tomatoes and beef, pork and apples, pineapple and pork, lemon and fish, and cheese and tomato. Chicken seems to go with almost any fruit. Mango, pineapple, and papaya, while sour fruits, are also especially helpful in tenderizing meat or aiding in the digestion of fish due to their enzyme content. Papaya contains papain; pineapple contains bromelain; and mango contains mangiferin. These are all enzymes that specialize in breaking down protein. Salsa, chow-chow, and other condiments also function as digestive aids for meats, beans, and peas.

Fermentation provides another type of sour taste. Nature ferments fruits and dairy products as a matter of course, but the earliest intentionally fermented foods were beer, wine, and cultured dairy products. Fermented vegetables provide a sour taste, good bacteria, and enzymes that aid in the digestion of meats and grains. For example, cabbage is fermented in several cultures around the world. In Germany, sauerkraut is eaten with heavy meats such as pork and beef. On the other hand, in Korea, kimchi is eaten with rice. If we look at traditional foodways, we can find many other examples such as pickles with cheese, chutney with either cheese, beans, or meat, and chow-chow with peas and beans.

It's important for the air-dominant person to take in adequate amounts of protein, and that requires adequate digestive juices. Sour foods can help improve digestion capability and food breakdown, which helps increase absorption of nutrients. Air folk should also try to avoid eating spoiled food, food that has been sitting out too long, and too many fermented foods. While fermented foods can be useful for digestive health, too many can overwhelm the small intestines with bacteria. Even good bacteria can cause issues in excess.

Neurotransmitters and Hormones

Protein is used in the manufacture of some hormones and neurotransmitters, such as thyroid hormone, adrenaline, endorphins, serotonin, oxytocin, and dopamine. Of particular importance to air people are the hormones linked to fight-or-flight, the stress hormones—adrenaline, cortisol, norepinephrine—and the role of the sympathetic nervous system in fight-or-flight. Air folk are especially susceptible to the effects of stress and are quick to react to stressful situations. They are prone to adrenal exhaustion, also called nervous exhaustion or cortisol dominance.

Early man dealt with many environmental stresses to survival that triggered fight-or-flight, such as facing a threatening animal, protecting hunting grounds or the tribe, or the uncertainty of food gathering and storage. There was also the thrill of the hunt itself. These are examples of acute stress, the stress of the moment.

For modern man, acute stressors still happen, but not as often and from very different sources. Chronic stress is more common, from too many hours at the office with too many deadlines, unattainable expectations in personal relationships, or how to make enough money to support a family. These examples of chronic stress have no clear endpoint. We don't know when that particular stress might end. Regardless of the source, whether acute or chronic, the body's reaction is the same.

In fight-or-flight, our body must decide whether to stand and fight, flee, or freeze. Which action is best for survival? That's a key question. If the threat is viewed as a challenge, then fight is the decision. If the threat is viewed as loss of control, then flight is the decision. Both are utilized in acute types of stress. On the other hand, if the situation is viewed as hopeless and unending, then freeze is the decision. The freeze mechanism is based on the belief of defeat and is the most common in chronic stress. Both fight and flight activate the release of adrenaline, but freeze also activates the release of cortisol. Let's look at this a bit closer.

When adrenaline is released, our heart rate goes up. Blood moves into our extremities and away from the digestive tract, readying our body for the physical action of fight or flight. All of our five senses intensify, especially sight and hearing. After the first rush of adrenaline and in order to maintain the stress reaction, the body releases cortisol to maintain the high-alert status.

All of this is taking place with the aid of the nervous system. It's the sympathetic nervous system that senses the danger and signals the brain to start the fight-or-flight process. This is wind in action. In acute stress, the sympathetic nervous system engages and stays on alert until the danger has passed, and then the parasympathetic nervous system aids in relaxing the body and mind. The stimulation to the sympathetic nervous system directly releases the stress hormones epinephrine and norepinephrine.

In chronic stress, the sympathetic nervous system stays on continual alert; it never takes a break—ever. Even when the danger has passed, it is still on alert thanks to cortisol. Cortisol takes longer to be secreted than the other stress hormones because it is released by the brain. It may take months for the mind to receive the signal that the threat is no longer there and reduce the levels of cortisol and stress hormones, and then the body must recover and repair.

Air people under stress often find it hard to eat; the appetite just goes away. Here they must be careful to continue eating some protein, or the body will begin using muscle for its needs.

During the stress cascade, glycogen is the preferred fuel. Once the stored glycogen from the liver and muscles is depleted, the body looks around for another source of fuel. That would be either fat or protein. It picks the one that converts the quickest because during stress the body needs energy quickly. The body would like to burn fat, but chronic stress stimulates production of a protein that reduces the body's ability to break down fat and so it uses protein instead.

Cortisol is a catabolic hormone that reduces protein synthesis, lowers the immune system, and prevents tissue growth. In other words, cortisol breaks down muscle for energy. Initially, the burning of muscle and the release of stress hormones will reduce the appetite and speed metabolism. Over time, in a chronic stress situation, cortisol will actually increase appetite and reduce metabolism, which causes weight gain. You can see this in air-dominant folks. First they lose weight and as the stress continues and they don't feel that it will ever end, then they start putting on weight, which often gives them a blown-up look. Thin air bones weren't meant to carry all that weight.

On a normal day, cortisol helps regulate our energy by selecting which type of fuel to burn, carbohydrates, fats, or protein. On a normal day, cortisol will signal the burning of fat, in the form of triglycerides, for fuel. But this isn't a normal day; this is another chronic stress day. Remember, cortisol is made from fat. And, the enzyme that converts inactive cortisone to active cortisol is found in fat tissue. The storage form of energy is fat, and cortisol directs fat storage deep into the abdomen to lay up fuel for the future—the future that has an uncertainty due to chronic stress. Cortisol is in complete control.

Air people are very susceptible to the effects of chronic stress because of the sensitivity of their nervous systems. Situations that wouldn't necessarily stress anyone else can send air into a stress cascade that lasts for days. In chronic stress, air folk are prone to emotionally blow up, yell, and say things they don't mean—in other words, throw a hissy fit. It's like letting the pressure off a valve. They've got to let it out and then it blows over.

Because of their sensitive natures and nervous systems, air people may appear standoffish, egotistical, or self-important. It's really the way that air people have of protecting themselves from the never-ending assault on their nervous systems. If it's out in the airways, air folk can pick it up, and for this reason, often appear psychic. They hum the song that's playing on the radio as they turn on the radio. They flip on the light switch and blow a bulb. They know what you are going to say as you say it.

Going to the mall or being around large crowds of people frazzles their nerves. They do better in smaller groups or in groups over which they have some control. For this reason, air folks make good professors, researchers, and writers.

Think about the role of stress and protein and the nervous system and the mind/body connection as we discuss the traits of air people. Chronic stress causes the body to burn protein for energy and store fat. Air people have a very sensitive nervous system and mind/body connection. For air people, any type of stress can quickly send them into an emotional tailspin.

Air Traits

Air people carry and move things too. They like to gather information and disperse it to the world in some manner. They analyze. They put their thoughts and ideas into words and send them out in the form of writing, research, poetry, or song. They want to know how people think and spend time thinking about this.

Air people are extremely concerned about what is fair and right. Often they advocate for social justice; they want to help make the world a better place. As rabble rousers or social analysts, air people help create the reform movements that make changes in society. They don't tend to be the leaders of the movement.

but prefer to work in more supportive roles, cranking out the words, the writings, or the speeches that support the cause. Think Bob Dylan, Allen Ginsberg, Yeats, Sartre, and Harriet Beecher Stowe. Air at its finest working for change. However, air people who really believe that change is needed and that they can help effect that change may become politicians. When the air is up but controlled, these folks can be very charismatic.

Air folks are smart and intellectual, and do well in their chosen professions as long as they stay on track. Sometimes, their intellect creates a barrier between them and others, and they often purposely create this barrier in order to protect their sensitive nature. Air folk are so sensitive and highly strung that it's very easy to hurt their feelings. Remember, they are running on nervous energy. Behind the facade of self-importance that is used as a defense is a quiet, lonely, sensitive soul who both loves and hates people at the same time. Who both needs and is repulsed by people at the same time. Who doesn't mind spending time alone to avoid making deeper emotional connections. These are the folks who treasure their true friends deeply and will be loyal even in times of adversity or absence.

Air people focus much of their thought around themselves, what affects them, but at a macro level. They think that what is good for them personally must be good for everyone. "I think therefore I am," said Descartes, a perfect example of air thought. At the same time, air people don't want to get too deep into their own thoughts, into their own psyche, because they might have to do something about themselves if they did. They seek answers to life's questions, but don't really know what to do with the info once they have it.

The mind of an air person is always busy, or at least engaged. They often have music playing in the background or the television on or the earbuds in. This background noise is a way of filtering out unwanted stimuli so they can continue thinking their thoughts. Sometimes, air people need this background noise just to fall asleep. Sound moves on air and certain noises, both real and imagined, often keep them awake.

Air people are the folks at parties who hide in the library waiting for someone to find them and have a good chat. They much prefer this one-on-one engagement instead of making small talk. Or they are the folks at parties who won't shut up and are the obnoxious motormouths who drive people crazy. Air people have trouble being social and have little regard for the niceties and compromises inherent in any relationship, including personal ones.

Air people don't like being needed by others, and they don't want others to depend upon them. That's a huge responsibility that forces air into a box or a mold. They want to love and be loved, but on their terms, and not society's or anyone else's. Air folks often go for unconventional relationships that seem conventional from the outside. Once they commit, they are devoted partners and parents, but still need some semblance of freedom, or at least the appearance of freedom. Air people want to be loved and may go through several relationships before finding the one person that understands them. If there is any strife in the relationship, air may be quiet for a short time, hours or days, and then will want to talk about it in great detail, often while walking.

Because air people love and need their freedom and flexibility of action and movement, they often work for themselves or work from home. Air people tend to have several jobs over their careers and tend to pick careers that offer the most flexibility and freedom.

Air people can appear aloof or unfriendly because they can be quite shy. Unfortunately, people do get on their nerves and for this reason, they can only take folks in small doses. Once you get to know an air person and they relax and feel safe around you, they can be quite interesting conversationalists. Since air people are avid readers and gatherers of information from many sources, they can converse on almost any topic.

Just as fire people need to connect with folks who have the same drive, passion, and *will* as they do; just as water people need to connect with like-minded others who *believe* as they do; air people need to connect with other like-minded people who *think* as they do. For air, it is all about the thought, the idea, the philosophy, the mind. Think of a flock of birds. All moving together, all thinking together. Or think of a computer club, everyone gathering together and sharing information but working on their own project. For water people, it's about relationships; for fire people, it's about the project or goal. But for air, it's about the idea. For example, fire will be in lust; water will be in love; and air will be in love with the idea of love.

Air people have a tendency to surround themselves with books, magazines, computers, file cabinets, and newspapers. Once the bookshelves are full, the books and magazines make little piles around the house. It's amazing how many air people have a filing cabinet at home with old newspaper or magazine articles neatly filed away along with their income taxes and other papers. Air people don't notice that others don't see their dusty mounds of information in quite the same way they do. They think their mess is not really messy since they know where to find anything. On the other hand, air folks want their surroundings to be clean, even if not neat, and will judge other people by how clean they keep their habitats.

For air people, thought manifests in words, whether verbal or written. For this reason, air people make excellent reporters, authors, editors, scientists, gamers, and computer experts. Air is also about communication, whether it's communication of the brain to the body through the nervous system or the communication of ideas and information to others, or the sending of information over the digital airways. Air is also about providing oxygen to the tissues for the production of energy.

Air needs direction to accomplish. Moving in a direction and maintaining that direction keeps air people focused and on task. Otherwise, they get sidetracked by other thoughts, ideas, or conversations. Fire needs a goal to fuel their passion; water needs boundaries to maintain good relationships; and air needs direction to stay in focus.

Regardless of your constitution, you are affected by air.

Excess Air

Excess air is overstimulation. There is so much stimulation that it's hard to focus and there are too many thoughts. But the stimulation is also very exciting and feeds on itself. As the stimulation shifts and air begins to calm, the air person will seek ways to bring it back up. The stimulation is addicting and air people enjoy this excess, but not for long periods of time. Too long in excess is exhausting and debilitating.

A common reason for excess air is stress, especially the stress associated with work or school and project deadlines. Staying up late at night drinking coffee and working are appealing up to a point. Then, rigidity of action and person sets in, soon followed by exhaustion. The physical effects of not eating enough, losing muscle, drinking too much caffeine, or smoking cigarettes begin to have a detrimental effect. It's time for the air person to slow down and ground themselves.

If this excess continues, the ability to follow a thought to a conclusion will be greatly impaired. Now we have the person who is flighty, has their head in the clouds, needs grounding, is an airhead, and someone who needs to come up for air and get a grip.

Attention deficit disorder (ADD) or attention-deficit/hyperactivity disorder (ADHD) are examples of excess air—too much input and the inability to filter unwanted thoughts or stimuli and focus. In this situation, an air child will seek caffeinated soft drinks, candy bars, or junk food. This quick rush of energy momentarily increases air, not lowers it. But air calls to air, and the more airy a person becomes, the longer they like to stay in that condition and the faster the mind turns. But stimulating substances can also increase concentration. Peppermint or spearmint tea is excellent to help an air person in this way.

The air adult will drink coffee to keep the air moving during the day, forget to eat or purposely avoid eating because it will ground and relax them, and then drink alcohol or smoke pot at night so they can sleep. That's too much stimulation. At this point the caffeine isn't stimulating the mind anymore, but is still stimulating the body and nervous system. Now, the air person still can't think, but can't sleep either. If the overstimulation continues, nervous exhaustion, or adrenal fatigue, is not far behind, and other opportunistic disorders, often autoimmune, may appear. In excess air, thoughts can become circular and so can emotional responses.

The state of excess air is an excited one. Folks are running on their second wind—going, going, going or talking, talking, talking. If they sit and relax for a moment, they might fall asleep. And when talking, they often jump from one topic to another without letting anyone else contribute to the conversation.

Excess air wants to move, move, move. These folks tend to wiggle in their chairs, get up and walk around, can't sit still, and twist and turn. All this wiggling and moving can take place while they are sleeping and may express as a type of restless leg syndrome.

Ever been around a person who just can't stop talking and you can't get a word in edgewise? When they leave, even though you haven't said anything, you are exhausted. You are wiped out. They've sucked out all your air.

A caution: People with excess air have a tendency to throw things when irritated. They usually throw objects on the ground, out the door, or at the wall, but not at people. They also like to throw around words. This can be quite disconcerting to experience. This may appear like fire, but it's just wind blowing. Contrast this to a fire person with temper—they will throw objects at you and the object could be their fist.

On the physical level, excess air is drying. Folks will be thin, dry, underweight, with long, stringy muscles. People with excess air are prone to food allergies and sensitivities, leaky gut syndrome, and sensitivities to chemical and environmental toxins, digestive disorders related to nerves, such as irritable bowel or ulcers, and disorders of the nervous system.

They are also prone to histamine reactions. Rashes, red spots, and hives are not uncommon, as excess air can carry heat. Blood sugar may be prompting the excess air person to reach for the sugar fix or more caffeine.

Folks with excess air should be cautious about the nightshade family; potatoes, tomatoes, eggplant, and green peppers may not digest well or contribute to inflammation. Histamine reactions tend to create an acidic stomach. During high-histamine times, foods and beverages that are acidic should be eaten with caution, such as tomatoes, vinegar, wine, fruit juices, and coffee. In the same vein, air children may exhibit redness around the mouth after eating acid foods such as pizza or spaghetti.

Nervine herbs, adequate protein with balanced carbohydrates from vegetable sources such as root vegetables, avoiding caffeine and processed sugar, and restful sleep will go a long way to restoring balance. Sleep and rest are extremely important to restore air. Also, the air person should avoid listening to the news, turn off the computer at least a couple of hours before bed, and avoid adrenaline-pumping movies late at night. A good book is therapeutic.

Because there is a tendency toward dryness, moistening herbs and foods can be helpful. Moistening foods include soups and stews, dairy products, cooked fruits, dried beans cooked well-done, and tender meats. Sweet and grounding well-cooked root vegetables such as carrots and winter squashes are also an excellent choice.

Sweet, moistening herbs such as angelica, anise, cooked burdock, fennel, red clover, mimosa, oatstraw, peach leaf, and sarsaparilla are useful.

Nervine herbs to help bring down excess air include skullcap, hops, wild lettuce, California poppy, passionflower, wood betony, peppermint, and valerian.

Deficient Air

Deficient air looks a bit like earth. Instead of the stimulation and excitation of excess air, in deficient air, there is sluggishness and over-relaxation. Depression could be a problem, along with blood sugar issues. In deficient air, there is a tendency to gain weight, stop moving or exercising, and become a bit of couch potato.

One cause of deficient air is that these folks feel that the world has turned against them or that they are alone in the world and no one likes them. Air people may not always want to be around other people, but they always want to be liked. Deficient air doesn't feel victimized the way a water person might, but their self-esteem certainly takes a hit. In this scenario, the deficient air person becomes reclusive and even more withdrawn.

There is nothing more demoralizing to an air person than someone questioning or not believing the air person's information. Questioning what an air person knows is a sure way to hurt their feelings, and this is like a blow to their gut. It immediately demoralizes them and takes away their energy. They feel drained, tired, and just want to be alone. If air stays deficient too long, they will lose interest in the world at large.

Deficient air shows a lack of ambition and motivation. There is reduced ability to communicate with people and more time is spent reading, writing, working on the computer, or playing video games. The shy air person becomes even more shy. They feel left out and alone and sort of shut down. Instead of sharing their information or sharing their writing, in deficiency state, they tend to keep it to themselves, hoarding information like Midas hoarded gold.

Deficient air people may exhibit jealousy, hoard information, and be critical of others. They may also exhibit selfishness in sharing their feelings or sharing their material possessions.

On a physical level, deficient air may manifest as weight gain, bloating, high blood sugar, high blood pressure, headaches, and mental sluggishness. Herbs and foods to balance blood sugar are extremely helpful. This person should also avoid any type of processed sugar, processed grains, or artificial sweeteners.

If air is deficient, it important to get the person up and moving. Air has to move to be healthy and happy. It's finding the balance that is important. Any type of exercise can be helpful with deficient air—walking, jogging, dancing, or any form of exercise that gives continuous movement.

Herbs to stimulate air include American ginseng, cayenne, elderberry, raspberry, gotu kola, hibiscus, lemon verbena, bay, pine, rose hips, huckleberry leaves, and sumac.

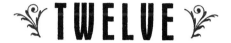

❧ TWELVE ❧

Earth: Sweet Blood

We could have saved the Earth but we were too damned cheap.

—Kurt Vonnegut

MRS. PRIDMORE WAS a local herbalist and fire-blower. She helped people with herbs, sound nutritional advice, a commonsense approach to affairs of the heart, and she could blow away the pain of fire. In her day, there was hardly anyone overweight or diabetic; it just wasn't the norm. Those few people who were overweight were often joked about and considered to be lazy or gluttonous. At best, they had a glandular disorder. While we might think this is a totally inappropriate view today, in Mrs. Pridmore's time, this was the common view. Most all the folks were farmers, hunters, and loggers, poor people who worked the fields, and folks whose gardens were their basic source of food. The effort of living was physically grueling and demanding. If you were overweight, you couldn't pull your share of the work on the farm. If you were overweight, you didn't have the stamina for those long, long days of hard work. And since everyone was so very poor and there was so little food to go around, if someone was overweight in a family, then there was a good chance that another family member wasn't getting enough to eat. This situation affected everyone. Also, folks who were overweight tended to be "city folk," people who didn't have to use their bodies in labor.

Being overweight could cause diabetes and was commonly recognized as so. However, there was another type of diabetes, the kind that caused weight loss, that was also commonly recognized as more serious and life-threatening. This was considered a serious health issue and acknowledged as a glandular problem that required medication. Today, we know that either type 1 or type 2 diabetes can cause weight loss, but it wasn't common knowledge in those days.

Even if a person thought they might have high blood sugar, few could afford a doctor's visit. There was a quick and easy home test that could infer, if not assess, how much sugar a person might have in their blood. If positive, it certainly warranted scraping the money together for a trip to the doctor.

Mrs. Pridmore would have folks pee into a pint fruit jar, and she would then sniff and check for a sweet smell. Urine with a sweet smell can indicate excess glucose that has spilled into the urine because there was more glucose than the kidneys could reabsorb. Ketones can also cause a sweet smell in the urine and could indicate that the body is burning fat for fuel. Regardless, urine with a consistently sweet smell should be investigated.

If Mrs. Pridmore had any doubts of the urine's sweetness, she would take the urine outside, weather permitting, and pour it on the ground where she knew the ants would find it. She had a piece of sandstone that she kept just for this purpose. Then she'd wait for the ants to arrive. And they almost always did. She liked to show folks how the ants swarmed their pee. It's quite disconcerting to see how the ants come swarming for the liquids from your body.

In a healthy body, there should be little or no glucose in urine, though the amount might be so low as to be considered not harmful. However, just drink twelve ounces of your favorite soft drink, or eat a chocolate fudge ice cream sundae, or drink five glasses of sweet tea and eat an extra helping of cobbler and see what happens. That's pretty much guaranteed to throw some sugar into the urine. It doesn't mean that the person is diabetic—only detailed medical testing can make that determination—but temporary rises in blood sugar after meals aren't uncommon.

So Mrs. Pridmore would show the person how the greedy ants would swarm over the sweet urine. And she would tell them a story while they stood there and watched the spectacle of the piss ants. One of her favorites was about Coyote, who was walking in the hot sun one day. He was getting hotter and hotter, and his tongue was hanging out his mouth. Coyote asked for a cloud to cool him off. So a little cloud came and covered Coyote's head. But Coyote wasn't satisfied, so he asked for a little rain to cool him off and quench his thirst. So the cloud began to rain. But Coyote still wasn't satisfied and he asked for more rain and then more. And pretty soon, it was pouring. And before Coyote knew it, the rain had washed him right away. And because of his greed, no one ever saw Coyote again. And all the while the piss ants swarmed over the urine. Folks generally got the message.

All About Earth

There are several definitions for earth. It is the planet on which we live, sometimes called Mother Earth. Here is our home, the land of our ancestors, and the land of our children. No other location in the vast array of planets and stars in the universes will ever be as hospitable to human beings as the one on which we already live. Planet Earth is perfect for us.

Earth is the dry part of the globe, the place where humans can build homes and towns. It is the soil beneath our feet. Rich, loamy soil fills the nostrils with the smell of fertility and brings the yearning to plant something, just anything in that hallowed ground. The word *earth* can also mean the ground beneath your feet. How solidly you plant your feet will depend on the type of ground on which you are standing. Burrowing animals go to earth or go to ground when hunted by either predators or humans.

The earth is full of minerals, rocks, dirt, and sand. These are the basic building materials for houses, buildings, and bridges, and the basic building materials of the human body. About 46 percent of the Earth's crust is made from oxygen, and silicon forms about 28 percent of it. The rest of the crust is made of sundry other minerals too numerous to mention. These surface minerals break down into smaller particles due to water and wind erosion and, along with certain microbes, become our soil. Here in this fertility, plants grow—the plants that feed, clothe, and shelter us.

Earth, then, is the inorganic minerals found both within the soil and deep within the planet, as well as the organic plant, animal, and human life that grows on the surface. It is the combination of both, as we are the combination of both.

Some people are rock hounds, amateur geologists, souring their local environments hunting and collecting rock specimens. Rock hounds often learn about the structure of rock formations and mineralogy in the process of rock collecting. Sedimentary rocks are made of sand, gravel, and shells that settle over time and harden; they often contain fossils. This is the most common rock where I live.

Metamorphic rocks are formed over time under the earth from intense heat and pressure. Igneous rock are formed from molten rock deep within the Earth.

And then, there is the definition of earth that most relates to our discussion in Southern Folk Medicine. Earth is one of the four elements in Greek humoral medicine and Southeast Native American folk medicine, as well as many other indigenous folk medicine systems around the world. Let's get started.

Types of Earth in the Body

Earth is cold by nature because it lacks movement. The temperature of the Earth is maintained by radiation from the sun, just as our temperature is maintained by our metabolism. There is a balance between the heat the Earth receives from the sun and the heat that is lost back to space. The human body certainly does the same, trying to maintain a balance between our internal temperature and the external temperature of the climate. We put clothes on or take clothes off to adjust our temperature. The Earth uses motion to also help balance temperature, and that includes rotation and revolution. While I might say that the Earth is static and cold, it's still a great ball spinning through space.

The Earth only heats while the sun is shining, and loses heat at night or on cloudy days. But the Earth doesn't heat evenly because about 70 percent of the surface is water. Soil and water heat at different rates, which causes uneven surface heating. Because the Earth is a sphere, and not a circle, the equator heats more than the poles. And because the Earth is spinning, we have seasons, which have different heating capabilities.

What about internal heat? We've all seen photos of volcanoes spewing massive amounts of molten lava, that's how continents are built. Because Earth was hot when it formed, there is leftover heat trapped inside. (This is actually a good illustration of how heat and inflammation can get trapped in the body.) This heat is being released to the surface, but is not the main contributor of the Earth's heat; that's the sun. The Earth continues to make some internal heat by radioactive decay of certain elements like uranium. The radioactive decay causes internal pressure to build, which leads to volcano eruptions and earthquakes.

The energy from the sun drives our weather on Earth, and the energy from the Earth builds mountains. It's a continual process that makes this world hospitable to all the life that lives on the surface of this planet. A change in either one of these sources of heat and humans are toast.

Where is earth in our bodies? Earth is actually one of the elements most easily seen, both visually and metaphorically, along with water. Earth is our supporting structure, our solidness, our house, our physical interface with the world. It is our bones, teeth, hair and skin, our nails, and our organs and glands. Place your hand on your opposite arm. Our earth is touchable and real.

Earth comprises most of the tissue in our body. It includes our musculoskeletal system—bones, muscles, and connective tissue, including ligaments, tendons, and cartilage. Earth in our bodies can also include any solid masses such as tumors, solid organs such as the liver, and glands such as the pancreas.

Think about how all the elements are coming together to create you, a unique human being. Earth is your structure; air the nervous system, breath, movement, and blood; water is all tissue fluids and gives shape to the physique; and fire is energy production, metabolism, and the activity of hormones. No element can work alone and, as you can see, no body system can either. We need the activities of all the different elements to be healthy, just like we need all the different body systems working together to be healthy. When everything is working in sync, we are in homeostasis.

Earth builds to form our structures. Cells come together to form membranes, which can cover the body, line the body, or divide organs into parts. An example would be the mucous membrane tissues that line the respiratory system, digestive system, gallbladder, bladder, and reproductive tissues. Tissues combine to form organs, which perform specific functions, such as the gallbladder storing bile. A group of organs come together to form systems that contribute to or share functions, such as the digestive system, the respiratory system, or the reproductive system.

All this begins with earth, with the basic building blocks. Let's begin this discussion of earth by looking at the types of tissue of which we are made: connective, epithelial, muscular, and nervous.

Connective Tissue

Let's start with the connective tissue, the most abundant of all tissues in the body and which is most commonly used for support and protection. Fat tissue is loose, connective tissue that stores energy. Both blood and lymph are specialized forms of connective tissue. And of course, cartilage and bone are dense connective tissue that give our foundation and support, form, stability, and ability to move. Some bones, like those in the rib cage, protect vital internal organs.

All tissues have an earth component. Let's look at some of these earthly components in greater detail.

BONES

Bone is the hardest of human tissue and the most enduring. It is tough and hard, and slow to decay. Fossils offer visual keys to our distant past, how our ancestors might have looked, and how they lived their lives. Bones dug from archeological sites offer a glimpse of the human age and experience on this planet. According to traditional knowledge, we inherit our bones, our foundation, from our fathers and our covering (skin and muscles) and our internal workings from our mothers. The bones of ancient man, our ancestors, are not dissimilar from our own.

Bones are often seen as a symbol of either mortality or death. Today, the skull and crossbones on a label are the symbol for poison or a warning of danger. In more ancient times, the symbol was a reminder of our mortality and the fleeting nature of human existence, and a reminder that the soul is immortal though the body is not.

Indigenous peoples used animal bones and shells for tools, weapons, musical instruments, and decoration. The study of the use of animal bones provides a unique glimpse into ancient societies and their culture and class systems. Tools made from bones include combs, sickles, daggers, digging sticks, fish hooks, needles, scrapers, and awls.

Because of their durability and seeming indestructibility, bones were given special magical powers by certain Indigenous tribes, as well as some Christian religions. Indigenous peoples used bones to make magical talismans. In the Catholic religion, bones have been viewed as religious relics and are believed to be imbedded with spiritual power that can be used by the owner of the relic. Sometimes the bones were painted or stained red in semblance of the life-giving properties of blood.

Throwing the bones or casting the bones was an ancient form of divination in some regions around the world, including North America, the Mediterranean, Africa, and Asia. In ancient Greece, temple priests used the anklebones of sheep (astragali), because they are more or less cube shaped, with four flat sides and two rounded ones; only the flat sides could be landed on. These were the forerunners of dice, which have been around for about 8,000 years. Dice were thrown to tell the future, and priests interpreted the message from the gods. About 7,000 years ago, the shape of the dice became more cube-like, and all six sides could be landed upon, which increased the potential for more complex outcomes. Throwing the dice became so popular that during a military campaign, Julius Caesar declared, "The die is cast."

Bone is active, living tissue and every ten years we replace worn-out bone with new bone in a process called remodeling. Our bones, and the minerals needed for their creation, form the framework for our bodies. Their strength and arrangement provide the support for our muscles and attachment points that give us our ability to walk upright and to turn, twist, jump, and run.

Bones support and protect softer tissues, store inorganic salts or minerals, and protect vital blood-producing cells in the marrow. Bones are named according to their shape—long, short, flat, and irregular. A bone's shape helps make possible its function.

Bone development begins during the first few weeks of life and continues into adulthood. Nutrients required for bone growth include vitamin D, which is necessary for the proper absorption of calcium. A lack of calcium in the bones of children is called rickets and in adults is called osteomalacia. The sun is our best source of vitamin D; however, supplementation may be necessary in some situations. In addition, vitamins A and C are also required for normal bone development. Hormones necessary for the production of bone include growth hormone, thyroxine, testosterone, and estrogen. Physical stress also stimulates bone growth, which is the reason exercise is vital to strong bones.

As we age, we begin to lose our earth, our structure, our bones. Bone loss begins about the age of thirty, and we proceed to lose about one-sixteenth of an inch a year thereafter. As we age, bones increasingly become susceptible to fracture due to loss of calcium and bone material influenced by the hormone-related changes of aging and our activity level. Although bone loss in men is slow and steady, bone loss in women is dramatically linked to changing hormones. However, by age seventy, both sexes are losing bone, losing earth, at about the same rate. We must work to maintain that structure with sound nutrition and weight-bearing exercises, and reduce diminishment as much as possible.

Sometimes the bone loss due to aging seems to happen all at once. On one visit to Grandma, she stands tall and straight, and then it seems that only a few months later she has suddenly shrunk. The diminishing of our house, our structure, seems to pertain to the spirit also. There is often less desire to travel, less desire to interact with social groups, and less willingness to start new ventures. As the structure diminishes, so does the Vital Energy.

JOINTS

Did you ever entertain your classmates at school by pulling your thumb down against your arm or otherwise contorting into weird shapes? If so, your genetics may have endowed you with hypermobility of the joints. But most of us have regular joint mobility.

A joint is the connection between the bones and muscles. That's a pretty simple definition, but a very important one. Wherever two bones meet, joints form. We have to have joints because bone doesn't bend. Joints allow skeletal muscles to move, enable bone growth, and are the reason parts of the skeleton are able to open, expand, and change shape at childbirth (temporary hypermobility). They also protect the ends of the bones from damage.

It's tendons and ligaments that create our joints and allow for the mobility of our bodies. They hold bone to bone in splendid perfection, which allows perfect function of the joint. Tendons, ligaments, and cartilage are all made from collagen and elastin in specific amounts for each tissue type.

Ligaments attach bone to bone and limit the movement of a joint to avoid dislocation or breakage. Because ligaments lengthen, they can overstretch. If that occurs, ligaments cannot return entirely to their original form. That's what happens during pregnancy when the uterine ligaments stretch to accommodate the growing baby but don't fully shrink to pre-pregnancy size or position. Or think about a sprained ankle, where the ligaments have overstretched due to injury and now the ankle is swollen and painful.

Tendons connect muscle to bone. Because tendons are elastic, they provide spring and release energy with movement, as well as resist tension. Overuse of tendons can result in tendinitis, such as tennis elbow, or carpal tunnel syndrome from repetitive movements.

Cartilage is stiffer than muscle and is found between the bones, at the end of the nose, outside of the ears, and in smaller respiratory tubes. Because cartilage does not contain blood vessels, it heals very slowly. Cartilage is supplied nutrients by compression that occurs with the pumping action of the cartilage that occurs with movement.

These are the tissues that make up the joints of the body. Although there are three types of joints in the body—fibrous, cartilaginous, and synovial—most of us are most concerned with synovial joints, which are the most common type of joint, or cartilaginous joints, which are found in the vertebrae of the spine. We depend upon the synovial joints for most of our movement. The ends of synovial joints are covered in a cartilage capsule, which is filled with synovial fluid to reduce wear and tear. The fluid not only lubricates but also supplies nutrients to the capsule. Folks who have back problems often have disk issues that have affected the cartilage between the vertebrae.

Dominant-earth folks tend to have wide, solid, and strong bones and are often blessed into the elderly years with good bones. Air, with the thinnest bones, is the most susceptible to age-related bone loss and must work at keeping bone strength and reducing loss. This is not so for earth folk, who are generally endowed with a solid framework that supports them for life.

Muscular Tissue

Muscles turn energy into motion. They pull us along, give us locomotion, and propel us through life. But they do more than that. Muscles allow us to express ourselves, communicate with others, and share ideas. Without the ability to move our arms, we can't paint a masterpiece. Without muscles, we can't talk, sing, or verbalize our thoughts and feelings. Without muscles, we can't fight or flee in times of danger or stress. Without our muscles, we are just a puddle of skin and bones.

Muscles are so important to our survival that they are highly specialized. Skeletal muscles provide movement, are under conscious control of our thoughts, and attach at bones. We can choose to pick up that penny. We can choose to walk around the block. We can choose to hug our friends and family members. Skeletal muscles can gain size and strength, then lose strength, and then gain it again, based on how often they are used and the purpose of their use. The type of exercise, movement, or work also determines how a muscle will respond to use.

Cardiac muscles, found only in the heart, are not under conscious control and not considered part of the musculoskeletal system. Their functioning is automatic to keep blood, oxygen, and vital nutrients circulating to our cells.

Smooth muscles are also not under conscious control; however, they are considered part of the musculoskeletal system. They help move fluids inside hollow structures or tubes such as those found in veins and arteries, the gastrointestinal tract, bronchial system, urinary tract, vagina, and within each individual cell. For example, the colon is a hollow tube that helps remove waste from our body in the form of feces. Although various life stresses may affect how the colon functions, such as stress, diet, hydration, and exercise regularity, it will generally empty at least once a day.

Every skeletal muscle is covered and separated from adjacent skeletal muscles by the amazing fascia, a dense connective tissue that separates and stabilizes muscles and organs. For the muscles, fascia reduces the friction of muscular force. Fascia is composed of the same material as ligaments and tendons, but is flexible and pliable; it moves as we move. It is a singular system—one large network that covers the whole body. If somehow we could only see the fascia, we could see how it wraps around the outside of each bone, how it encloses and separates each muscle and organ, how it forms the outline of the breasts. The only areas of the body either missing or limited in fascia are areas of the digestive tract, the respiratory system, and the lymph system. These tubes don't require fascia for support.

How do muscles move? Their movement is caused by an electrical stimulation (air) that travels through the nerves and contracts the muscle. Without the ATP (fire) created through cellular respiration, the muscles don't have the energy to move even with the electrical stimulation. During strenuous activity, the cardiovascular system may not be able to supply enough oxygen to the muscles to create more ATP, resulting in an oxygen debt and the formation of lactic acid.

Muscles contract to move, which is called a twitch. Slow-twitch muscle fibers produce enough ATP to contract for long periods. Fast-twitch muscle fibers contract more rapidly but fatigue quickly because they cannot generate ATP quickly enough. Which are you?

Earth folks tend to have strong, solid muscles that respond well to exercise activities such as weight lifting and aerobics. They are not usually the fastest runners (air), or most competitive athletes (fire), or the most creative yoga instructors (water), but respond well to a variety of exercise options. Weight lifting, bicycling, and square dancing would all uniquely satisfy an earth person's need for movement.

Epithelial Tissue

The most common epithelial tissue that we see is our skin. It covers the body's surface and acts as a surface barrier to keep out bacteria, viruses, and yeast. For this reason, it is a first line of defense.

The skin is waterproof, both keeping out water and at the same time minimizing internal water loss. It protects underlying structures such as the heart, blood vessels, muscles, nerves, and organs. The skin is a sensory organ that lets us touch and be touched and feel it. It helps regulate body temperature and helps us sweat out impurities. And most importantly, it helps us make just the right amount of vitamin D.

Epithelial tissue also forms the lining for most internal cavities and hollow organs, including the digestive system and other mucous membrane tissues. This is also the major tissue of glands. The function of epithelial tissue includes protection, secretion, diffusion, sensory perception, absorption, and filtration.

One of the hallmarks of epithelial tissue is that, as long as it receives good nutrition, it will repair and regenerate very fast. Another characteristic is that it contains no blood vessels but lots of nerve tissue. If you damage epithelial tissue, you might not bleed, but you'll sure feel it.

Nerve Tissue

The signals are sent and the signals are received. Nerve cells form the structure that carries information from the body to the brain and from the brain to the body. The role of the nervous system was discussed in detail in the chapter on air or sour blood.

Nerve cells form the basis of our five senses, which allow us to interface with our environment and with each other. There is a dedicated organ for each sense: eyes for sight; ears for hearing; tongue for taste; skin for touch; and nose for smell. These are the traditional senses, but there are lesser ones, including the sense of balance, temperature, kinesthetic sense, and pain. The sense of balance keeps us upright and not falling down every few minutes. As we age, many people begin to lose this sense and are more prone to falls. Continued physical activity and practice will help keep this sense strong. The sense of temperature helps us determine if the environment is hot or cold. When we touch a hot plate with our fingers, we immediately know that it is hot and painful, another of the senses. Kinesthetic sense helps us determine the weight of an object in our hands or one that we are about to pick up. It also helps us determine our body position and feel the relationship between parts of our body. The science of kinesiology has developed from the investigation into this sense.

The nervous systems of earth folks aren't as sensitive as those of their opposite, air. Dominant-earth people seem to have a really "thick skin" that offers protection from hurtful words uttered in the heat of the moment by loved ones. They are quite forgiving and patient with others, a trait the other three elements might cultivate.

Stem Cells

Every structure, every building, must have a blueprint for its design and instructions on how to put it together. In the human body, our blueprint is our DNA, our genetic treasury. But we also need the proper materials for the structure being built. Our bodies are no exception. For our bodies, the ultimate earth, the origin of every cell, the source of our structure, and the basic building material is the stem cell. Deep, deep in the body, totally protected by the strong walls of our bones, is the manufacturing facility of our cells—the bone marrow. Here, in this protected place, our bone marrow produces stem cells, which are young, immature cells, and turns them into the type of cell we need. From stem cells we make hair, skin, nails, muscles, bone, red blood cells, white blood cells, and complete organ systems. Whatever type of tissue we need, whenever we need it, the stem cell is ready and able.

The bone marrow is the soft and spongy tissue found in the hollow spaces in the interior of bones. If you've ever cooked roast beef, the fatty material in the center of the bone is the marrow. Indigenous peoples ate the fatty marrow from the cooked bone to make their bodies stronger and improve their fat intake because wild game often has very little fat. Cultures from around the world have recipes utilizing bone broth for both its tasty appeal and its contribution to good health. Bone broth is the latest superfood and can be found on grocery store shelves and in some restaurants.

In babies, all bone marrow makes stem cells; however, by the time we are adults, the active marrow is generally confined to the large bones such as the hips. There are two types of marrow: red marrow and yellow marrow. In babies, most all the marrow is red and produces red blood cells, white blood cells, and platelets. In adults, about half the marrow in the body is yellow and produces bone cells, fat, and cartilage. Neural stem cells have been found in the brain; epithelial stem cells in the lining of the digestive tract; and skin stem cells in the basal layer of the epidermis. Mesenchymal stem cells provide the connection between the circulatory, immune, endocrine, and nervous systems—the ultimate mind/body connection.

The stem cell is the progenitor of all our earth. It is a blank slate, an undifferentiated cell, and with just a signal, we turn that blank slate into the type of cell we need the most, whether bone, blood, or fat. It's a truly remarkable system and I am continually amazed by human physiology.

The Nature of Earth

Earth is associated with the humor or body fluid of black bile, the color black, and the taste of sweet. It governs structures in the body including the neck, throat, vocal chords, intestines, belly, abdomen, skin, bones, knees, skeletal system, and teeth. It also, to some extent, governs the structure of the glands, organs, and nervous system, as well as the structure of the blood vessels and lymphatic vessels. The earth element is also known as sweet blood in the Southern blood types.

Earth is composed of both organic and inorganic substances. Any substance in the Earth, such as minerals, fall under the domain of earth. Any plant growing in the soil falls under the earth element. Even salt is an earth mineral whose main action is on water. Our body takes the earth, metabolizes it, and creates living tissue. This is true of humans, or animals, and to some extent plants. There would be no food without the earth, no plants without the earth. With care and attention to food combining, most people can get all they need to be healthy from the earth. All our primary nutrients—fats, carbohydrates, and proteins—are available from the earth. There isn't a process in the body that isn't influenced by earth.

We've discussed in detail the role that earth plays in the body's structures, but there's more. To understand the nature of the earth element, it is important to understand the nature of carbohydrates and the taste of sweet, and how the body makes and uses energy from the point of view of the fuel and not the process (fire and air) as was discussed previously.

There has been some debate over the centuries concerning exactly what black bile might be. It has been described as consisting of poisons or toxins that are eliminated through the feces or urine. Or, it could be a deranged form of yellow bile that has visible blood in it. Alternatively, this type of bile might be the visible results of internal bleeding eliminated through any orifice. Some authors associate black bile with the gallbladder and others with the kidneys and spleen. Menstrual blood might also fit this description. Actually, any tissue breakdown could fit this description.

The body fluid associated with black bile is not as clearly distinguished as that associated with blood, yellow bile, or water. But the main disorder in Southern Folk Medicine associated with earth is sweet blood and its humor black bile is quite obvious: sugar in the blood, also known as diabetes. But more on that later.

I hope that you can continue to see the interrelationship of the elements in the body.

The Sweet Taste of Earth

The taste of sweet is one our most preferred tastes—just ask any child. It is the taste we all love and some crave. Our craving, our need for the taste of sweet, has led to wars, slavery, and obesity.

A sweet food in our mouth creates a bit of mucus on the tongue but relaxes the mouth and the whole body. This is one reason dessert comes at the end of the meal: It is relaxing and calming.

This is also the reason we sweeten cough syrups with sugar or honey; the taste itself is relaxing and, in a pinch, a bit of sugar water can often stop a cough. Another reason that the Western custom of dessert occurs at the end of the meal was due to limited access to sweeteners. Today that isn't an issue. Sugar is accessible, even overaccessible, to everyone, and we could have dessert all day long, but I don't think most people's digestion could handle it, nor would it be very healthy for the body.

Sweet is the taste of sugar, the taste of carbohydrates in food. It's the taste that lets our body know that the food will be a quick source of energy. It is naturally found as fructose in fruit or lactose in dairy products. Our ancestors had to work hard to capture this taste in food, but we don't; it's just a trip to the nearest supermarket.

Foods high in carbohydrates are the source of the glucose needed by the body to perform day-to-day activities. All carbohydrates have to be converted into glucose because this is the only form of sugar the body uses. The three types of carbohydrates we eat are sugar, starch, and fiber. The carbohydrates that contain sugars are classified as either simple or complex.

Simple carbohydrates, found in fruits, milk, vegetables, and processed foods, are broken down quickly for energy. Starches, found in peas, potatoes, and breads, are also turned into glucose. Complex carbohydrates, found in whole grains, root vegetables, fruits, and legumes, provide energy and are an excellent source of fiber. Lovely fiber makes us feel full quicker, helps moderate blood sugar and cholesterol, and helps keep the colon healthy and functioning properly.

Our ancestors had to work very hard for their food. It wasn't cheap, easy, and plentiful the way it is today. Fruits and root vegetables were the most common sweet foods among poor Western Europeans. Only the wealthy could afford honey or spices to sweeten their food. In the New World, fruits, sweet herbs, and maple syrup were the most common sweeteners used by Native Americans.

But all that changed when humans began cultivating the grass known as sugarcane and processing it into a form that could be easily transported. Originally native to Southeast Asia, the first recorded processing of sugarcane into crystals took place in India. The sugar crystals were tasty, sweet, and in great demand. European countries built vast numbers of plantations in the Caribbean, worked by African slaves, to grow and process sugarcane. When I was a child, here in Alabama, we grew our own sugarcane, and the men in the community came together in the fall to make cane syrup and molasses. I remember running barefoot on the grass sucking on a sliver of sugarcane. We also grew sorghum, a high-sugar grass from Africa, and made "homemade syrup" or sorghum syrup in the fall.

But let's not stop there. In our food culture, we are being overwhelmed with earth. In addition to honey, maple syrup, corn syrup, sorghum syrup, molasses, and table sugar, let's not forget all the other sources of sugar on the market, such as guava syrup, agave, rice syrup, barley malt, brown sugar, date sugar, beet sugar, palm sugar, coconut sugar, powdered fructose, apple syrup, and yacon sugar. We could also mention sweet herbs such as stevia and licorice, which can be easily added to sweeten beverages and other foods. Quite a list! And then there are the artificial sweeteners and sugar substitutes, aspartame, sucralose, and saccharin.

Humans definitely have a love affair with sweet. It is a taste that we crave, satisfying more than our energy needs. It's the taste most often eaten in times of stress and emotional distress. It's the taste of special occasions and celebrations, weddings, anniversaries, birthdays, and family reunions. Sweets are so important to us, so important to our taste and psyche, that we named a whole category of foods to honor them: desserts. The sweet taste of food and beverages has become our reward, emotional balm, and favored food, especially in times of unhappiness.

Because of our love affair with sweets and the inability of so many people to control their consumption, sweets have been blamed for obesity, poor health, poor eating habits, and poor teeth. But do keep in mind, there is a huge difference between eating foods with natural sugars, such as fruits and root vegetables, and eating foods made with processed sugars. The effect is very different in our bodies.

In general, earth constitution is drawn to sweet foods. These are the folks who can eat a doughnut and coffee for breakfast and have a good time. Not so for air and fire constitutions, or even water. These are also the folks who like a sweet snack before bedtime and keep cookies, cakes, pies, or ice cream handy for their sweet tooth. As long as earth people eat sweets in moderation and keep active, they may not experience any detrimental effects or excessive weight gain. They've just got to keep moving.

Producing Energy—Vitamin C, Citric Acid, and Glucose

We've discussed energy production by the Krebs or citric acid cycle in the chapters on fire and air, and now we'll continue the discussion here. It takes the influence of all three of these elements to produce the energy our body needs to function. This is a further illustration of the complexity and interaction of the elements. Carbohydrates drive the cycle, but fats and proteins are also required, as is, importantly, citric acid. And yes, it's the same citric acid that is found in citrus fruits, but we make our own. Don't confuse vitamin C and citric acid. Though they may be found together in foods, they are not the same thing.

Nutrients needed for the Krebs cycle include thiamin, riboflavin, niacin, vitamin C, pantothenic acid, vitamins B6, B12, and folate, calcium, magnesium, and trace minerals. Our bodies extract or make these nutrients from our food. One nutrient is especially vital in our diets because we can't store this nutrient for any length of time: vitamin C. We must have a steady supply for good health.

Most animals make their vitamin C from glucose, but not humans, bats, primates, or guinea pigs. We must receive this essential nutrient from our food. And it is essential because without adequate levels of vitamin C, we'll die, and pretty quickly—hard-core information to think about. The lack of vitamin C is called scurvy, which plagued sailors on long voyages, though any folks who are eating a highly processed diet or in a poor socioeconomic status might also be susceptible to a deficiency.

Our best sources of vitamin C are raw fruits and vegetables and fermented foods. Old-time mariners had to figure out a way to carry vitamin C–rich foods on long voyages, and fruits and sauerkraut were often the best choices. We can't store vitamin C for more than a few weeks, which means that at some point in the history of the human race, we had access to vitamin C–rich foods on a regular basis, which points to a tropical environment.

In nature, vitamin C and natural sugars are found together, and so fruit was our ancestors' first food choice for both of these vital substances. Vitamin C is needed to build connective tissue (earth), and signs of vitamin C deficiency can include bleeding gums, mouth ulcers, loose teeth, anemia, and lack of energy. All signs of deficient earth. The cardiovascular system has a high requirement for vitamin C, and a deficiency can lead to high blood pressure, easy bruising, and lax vessels, among other issues. Vitamin C can help prevent atherosclerosis and lower high cholesterol. The blood is just a very specialized form of connective tissue, and all connective tissue requires vitamin C. Also, without adequate levels of vitamin C, we have a poorly supported immune system with poor wound healing and reduced ability to fight off infection. Are you beginning to see how important this nutrient is to our health?

Vitamin C is an antioxidant, which plays a role in collagen and amino acid formation. It's required for the formation of stress hormones and helps us deal with stress in a healthier manner. Vitamin C can help reduce cholesterol levels and is needed for the uptake and utilization of iron. It helps keep vitamins A and E potent, and aids in the absorption of iron and calcium. Vitamin C helps vision in the elderly.

If vitamin C and glucose share a relationship, then so do vitamin C and insulin. Vitamin C follows insulin into a cell, much the same way that water follows salt. An important receptor activates in response to insulin to allow both glucose and vitamin C to enter the cell. Because glucose has a greater affinity for the insulin receptor, more glucose will enter the cell than vitamin C. If the person has high circulating blood sugar, then limited vitamin C enters the cell. Certain systems require high amounts of vitamin C for efficient operation, such as white blood cells. These cells have more insulin pumps than others in order to allow enough vitamin C into the cell to function as an antioxidant. If too much glucose is circulating in relation to vitamin C, then the cells won't have the antioxidant capacity needed. This is one way that high blood sugar reduces immune functioning. High blood sugar is excess earth in Southern Folk Medicine, and we'll talk more about this shortly.

But we need glucose, and ultimately, when pertaining to dietary intake, it's all about wise food choices. Glucose, from carbohydrates in the standard American diet based on processed sugar, is quick, easy, cheap fuel for most of the body's processes. Once a carbohydrate food has been digested, the resulting glucose goes from the small intestine to the liver and then enters the bloodstream to make its way around the body, providing immediate energy to needy cells. Once glucose leaves the liver and enters the bloodstream, it needs insulin, a protein hormone, to penetrate the cells. Without adequate insulin, glucose stays in the bloodstream and glucose levels rise. Beta cells in the pancreas monitor blood levels of glucose and signal the pancreas to produce insulin in response. Insulin is released from the pancreas into the bloodstream to unlock each cell to uptake glucose.

In addition, insulin stimulates muscle and liver cells to produce glycogen, the storage form of glucose. It also stimulates fat cells to make fats. And insulin stimulates the liver and muscles to make proteins from amino acids. Unlike fat, which can be stored in unlimited quantities, carbohydrates and proteins are fuels that the body can only store in limited amounts. Any glucose not immediately used or needed is taken to the liver for storage as glycogen. Any leftover glucose that can't be either used or stored is now stored as fat for future energy needs.

When food is scarce, as was often true in times past, the alpha cells in the pancreas produced another protein hormone, glucagon, to stimulate the liver and muscles to break down stored glycogen found there. Your body uses both insulin and glucagon in a carefully choreographed dance to maintain balanced levels of glucose in the blood and to fuel body processes.

According to Southern Folk Medicine tradition, fresh blood has a sweet taste because sugar is always in the blood. And depending on the health of the individual, there may also be undertones of iron in fresh blood. Because all blood is sweet, it is the degree of sweetness that becomes the issue. Excessively sweet blood is known as high sugar, high blood sugar, sugar in the blood and, in more recent times, diabetes. Modern medicine categorizes these disorders as insulin resistance syndrome, which is also called metabolic syndrome or syndrome X, or pre-diabetes. When the body has slowed its production of insulin or can't uptake what is made, this is known as type 2 diabetes. And when the body is no longer making insulin, this is known as type 1 diabetes.

Excessively sweet blood can have many causes. Traditionally, it was thought that high sugar came from eating too many sweets. For my relatives in the South, sweet blood came from a high-calorie diet filled with simple carbohydrates, high fat, and low protein: the diet of poor whites and blacks who worked the cotton fields and needed energy. Biscuit and gravy for breakfast; peas and cornbread for supper. This diet fueled immediate energy needs but left little for storage and provided no antioxidants and little protein. Some garden vegetables in season provided a definite benefit for health when it was possible to grow them. In some ways, the current standard American diet isn't much different from the diet of the cotton field workers and slaves. Too many simple carbohydrates, too much fat, too much salt, too much processed sugar, poor-quality protein, and lack of antioxidants from fresh fruits and vegetables.

Our sweet taste buds are generally satisfied with natural sweets found in root vegetables like winter squash, beets and sweet potatoes, sweet herbs, and fruits. Give these foods a try. They also contain natural antioxidants along with fiber to move the colon and improve elimination, and prevent the buildup of black bile.

Think about the nature of earth, sugar, and insulin as we discuss the traits of earth people. Both glucose and vitamin C follow insulin into a cell. All tissue production falls under the domain of earth and requires vitamin C for production. Earth is the element that affects all the others in some fashion. Fire burns on earth and may change organic material into its constituent components, but it doesn't destroy the solid earth. Water covers earth and causes stagnation, but doesn't destroy it. And air moves earth but doesn't destroy it. Earth is immobile, fixed, and steadfast.

Earth Traits

Earth people build. They might build a business, a garden, a house, or a relationship. They are prone to building great works of art. Whatever they choose to build, it will be done to the best of their ability—a true masterpiece. People with dominant earth love to understand and follow the steps within a process, while at the same time looking for ways to make the process more practical or work better. Whatever else, earth folks like things to be practical and useful.

Earth folk are survivalists in the true sense of the word. They'll follow the rules of society, believing that the rules are there for a reason and need to be enforced. When earth folk perceive that this is no longer true, they make preparations for the rules to be broken, but don't generally lead the charge to break the rules themselves, unless they are personally threatened. In that scenario, earth folks are also good at changing an unfair or unjust component of their cultural structure that is no longer working.

People with a dominant earth element are hardworking, stable, and generally grounded in reality. Common sense is their virtue. They have a calm and easygoing aspect to their personality and are seldom riled. These folks are methodical and understand that pacing is important.

Earth folks make loyal and steadfast friends. They don't make friends easily or quickly, and tend to cherish each friend or relationship they have. If the relationship turns sour, these folks will hold on and try to work it out instead of immediately giving up. They have tenacity and are reliable. They can be a bit predictable. which is both comforting and, occasionally, a bit boring.

Folks with dominant earth are cautious, and security is important to them. They need to feel secure emotionally, financially, and physically in order to do their best work. Earth people are concerned with amassing and gathering the things they need to feel secure. They are frugal with their money and like to keep some assets in savings or plan ahead financially for the future.

Earth folks innately understand structure, whether we are speaking of socio-economic structure, corporate structure, or the structure of the legal system. For this reason, they make good business people, lawyers, judges, and builders.

Earth is a fertile element, and whatever seed is planted, whether plant or human, tends to grow strong and straight. They also make excellent gardeners, landscape architects, groundskeepers, and forest rangers.

In addition to being good builders, Earth folk make good architects, engineers, mechanics, plumbers, and tradespeople of all professions. They like using their hands and can take delight in the outcome of their physical labor.

Earth is solid and immoveable, and earth people can also be quite stubborn and immovable once they've made up their minds. And once they've made up their minds, earth people are generally not open to hearing new information on the topic. It might take an earth person weeks to investigate and research something before making a decision, especially on major purchases.

Earth people are very aware of class structure and understand the importance of status within their culture. They are adept at moving up the social and economic ladder, whether it's within a corporate structure or a social structure.

Earth people can be very creative, especially as writers of fiction, poets, and painters. They have the innate ability to complete their projects, an excellent trait that is sometimes missing in fire and air elements. As authors, they do well writing a series of books building on a theme, or world-building. Earth folks work at their craft or their art and only get better with age. These are the old masters who create masterpieces, as opposed to the shooting stars who are here and gone.

They are physically strong and very sturdy, with wide and strong bones. Earth people need to move to be healthy. Without movement, they don't burn excess carbohydrates and tend to accumulate belly fat. People with a strong earth element tend to gravitate toward lifting weights, but a cardiovascular component in their exercise program is very important to their overall health. Alternately, earth people do well in professions that are physically demanding such as construction and landscaping, which allow their fairly constant movement throughout the day.

Earth people are prone to depression and seasonal affective disorder, and regular exercise also helps them maintain a good mood and avoid the winter blues. These are the folks that find that a little serotonin really boosts their mood. For this reason, they often do well during times of stress or during the winter with St. John's wort.

Earth people must be especially diligent in the avoidance of too many simple carbohydrates and not enough complex carbohydrates. It's quite easy for an earth person to be drawn to eating processed grains in white breads, cakes, pies, cookies, cobblers, pasta, crackers, and white rice. These foods provide earth people with quick energy when their own daily allotment is running low. It becomes a vicious cycle: eat, feel more energetic, feel tired; eat, feel more energetic, feel tired.

Earth people have a limited amount of energy to fuel their day's activities even when eating healthy. The day is over, their work is done, and they are ready for rest and recreation, and with good reason—they need it. A good night's sleep will replenish their energy levels, and they will be ready for a new day of work. Even though earth folks like to socialize, sometimes they are just too tired but should make the effort. Remember the adage, "All work and no play makes Jack a dull boy."

Fire people have *will,* water people *believe,* air people *think,* and earth people *analyze.*

Excess Earth

Excess earth can present in the personality as hoarding, which is fueled by fear of some kind: fear of losing a job, fear that the government will fail, fear that there won't be enough for old age, or fear that they can't support the family structure. In excess earth, hoarding goes to the extreme, and people hoard articles like cardboard boxes, straws, plastic utensils, or newspapers and magazines. They start hoarding items with limited uses. This can become a psychological illness.

Earth people are very concerned with security and having all the "things" they need to be safe and secure. When earth is out of balance to the excess, enough is never enough. There is never enough food in storage or guns in the cabinet. Life becomes about having enough money, food, tools, computers, cars, and televisions. It is the having of physical possessions that becomes an unhealthy drive. The packrat becomes the hoarder.

People with excess earth may also become jealous, possessive, and insecure of their possessions and their relationships. At the extreme excess, they will destroy what they love to keep anyone else from having it. In excess, earth can move into extreme conservatism and feel threatened at every turn. Normally, earth people follow rules and regulations to the letter and will not bend or break them, but excess earth will break the rules in the name of survival. They also become very tight-fisted, miserly, and stingy. In excess, earth people withhold donations from charities, as well as family and friends.

Physically, excess earth can present as thick and sweet blood or diabetes. There is a tendency toward metabolic syndrome, pre-diabetes, and diabetes, obesity, and high blood pressure. There is fatigue and loss of energy and enthusiasm— the perfect couch potato. Parasites may become a problem due to unhealthy eating habits, sweet blood, and lack of movement or exercise. Depression, insecurity, and isolation may become an issue. There is a tendency to self-medicate with sweets and other simple carbohydrates and to snack between meals. Excess earth may also present with thyroid issues, lymph stagnation, fibroid tumors, fibrocystic breasts, and cancerous tumors. Too much earth may also present as bursitis, stiffness in the joints, tight muscles, and arthritic conditions.

Herbs to help bring excess earth back into balance include American ginseng, dandelion, sarsaparilla, sumac, huckleberry leaves, hawthorn, hibiscus, juniper or cedar berries, blueberry leaves, and holy basil.

Deficient Earth

People with Deficient Earth may appear to have a touch of air element. They may be a little jittery, self-centered, and overly confident. Deficient earth may take on a veneer of self-importance and overindulge in purchases such as clothes, furniture, and electronics, buying the best and most expensive instead of only what they need. Their normal frugality goes out the window because their awareness of status is heightened. They don't really need it but buy it anyway. In deficient earth, folks become concerned about wearing the latest fashions, how many computers they own, or what type of vehicle they drive. But this behavior can't last, and once the credit card is filled, a major adjustment is needed.

Their earthy common sense is replaced by foolishness and impracticality. For example, in the area of romance, deficient earth may start stalking the object of their affection. Their insecurity may drive them to make false accusations against their partners that have no basis in truth. Being deficient in earth, the fear of losing something precious, actually causes them to push away those they love with their behavior. Deficient earth people can also make hateful, hasty, and nasty comments to those they love the most.

Deficient earth is prone to low blood sugar or hypoglycemia. In addition, there is a tendency for digestive problems, especially in the colon. Constipation, slow or incomplete evacuation, and a bloated small intestinal area may be present. Deficient earth folks may appear nervous and anxious in normal situations. The liver and spleen may also be deficient in function.

People with deficient earth may also have a tendency toward sciatica, lumbago, and tingling in the hands and feet. There may also be muscle spasms, tics, and Tourette's syndrome.

Foods high in good complex carbohydrates are good choices—root vegetables, fruits, and whole grains. These same foods work well for excess earth also.

Herbs that can help bring balance to deficient earth are American ginseng, sarsaparilla, angelica, cornsilk, fennel, fenugreek, honeysuckle, red clover, alfalfa, oatstraw, peach leaf, Solomon's seal, skullcap, and passionflower.

❧ THIRTEEN ❧

What's Your Constitutional Makeup?

HERE IS A short questionnaire to help determine your constitutional makeup. Please remember that we are a combination of all four elements, though we might have one element that is dominant. There are many combinations of your elemental makeup that can occur. No combination is right and no combination is wrong. You are what you are, a unique and vital human being.

After you have finished the quiz, reread the sections on the constitutions that are most applicable to your unique makeup.

Directions

Please answer each question to the best of your ability, thinking about how you are feeling now, the circumstance of today. Don't think about how you were ten years ago or in your childhood. It's about now.

1. Number a piece of paper from 1 to 20.

2. Write the letter—A, B, C, D in answer to the question.

3. When finished, add up the number of As, Bs, Cs, and Ds.

4. Check the answer key at the end of the questionnaire to understand your constitution.

Questions

1. Which of the following best describes your facial features? (It's OK to look in a mirror or ask a friend.)

    A. Broad forehead, sparkly eyes, narrow or square jaw and chin

    B. Rounded forehead and face, small mouth and straight teeth, rounded chin

    C. Heart-shaped face, forehead narrowing at top, small mouth, crowded teeth, pointed chin

    D. Oval or square face, high forehead, open eyes, wide, even teeth and mouth, broad chin

2. Which of the following best describes your basic skeletal structure? (It's OK to ask a friend if unsure.)

    A. Medium build and boned, athletic, well-defined muscles

    B. Medium build and boned, strong, but less-defined muscles

    C. Narrow build, long-limbed, fine-boned, long muscles

    D. Wide build, solid, thick-boned, may carry a few pounds

3. Where do you notice weight changes first?

    A. Abdomen, midriff, upper arms, butt

    B. Mostly all over, but especially breasts and stomach area

    C. Stomach area, upper thighs, waist, abdomen

    D. All over but especially face, arms, thighs, calves

4. What happens when you get really angry?

    A. Becomes controlling, shows temper, gets physical, then cries

    B. Cry, pout, complain, get emotional, and raise voice

    C. Say ugly words, throw things, blame, stomp off, slam doors, isolate

    D. Walk away, deny the situation, sulk, withdraw, and then later accuse, blame

5. Which do you do when you get good news?

   A. Want to share excitement, get others excited, plan big things

   B. Exclaim, laugh, want to be with close family and friends, but no celebration

   C. Want to be with people, throw a party and be the center of attention

   D. Want to celebrate, go out to eat with family and friends, get a burst of creative energy

6. What happens when someone you don't know says something nasty to you?

   A. Lose temper and say something childish back, can become physical

   B. Have hurt feelings and tear up

   C. Either respond with sarcasm and smart attitude or feel shocked and nervous

   D. No immediate response, then stew on it later

7. What snack food do you grab during times of stress?

   A. Salty or greasy foods such as chips, nuts, dried meat

   B. Ice cream, yogurt, cheese, fruit, or whatever is left over in the fridge

   C. Sandwiches, soup, or junk food

   D. Cookies, cake, bread, sugary desserts

8. What is your favorite type of exercise?

   A. Competitive sports and activities; like to be the trainer or group leader

   B. Group activity as participant or noncompetitive activities like hiking or dance

   C. Walking, jogging, yoga but likes freedom to create own program

   D. Needs variety to stay engaged, needs structure, weight lifting, endurance training

9. What is your favorite method of learning?

   A. Learn by watching others or using pictures or images

   B. Learn by using sound or music; learn in groups

   C. Learn by teaching others; learn by using words

   D. Learn by hands-on practice; learn by doing

10. What is your preferred language of showing love to others?

    A. Physical touch

    B. Acts of service and devotion

    C. Words of love and affirmation

    D. Gift-giving; spending quality time together

11. What would be the characteristics of your ideal occupation?

    A. Managing a team, leading an organization, working on a project

    B. Helping people, service work, care professions

    C. Academics, researcher, communications, writer

    D. Building, agriculture, creating a masterpiece

12. Which of the following is your idea of success?

    A. A project well done, contributing to your profession, being all that you can be

    B. Good relationships, rewarding family life, active community or church member

    C. Doing something that helps others, writing a book, setting an example for others

    D. Getting the most out of life, having a good retirement, living an ethical, balanced life

13. Which would be your ideal sleep cycle and pattern for the day?

   A. Don't need a lot of sleep, jump up ready to go, power nap when needed

   B. Need lots of sleep and sleep routine, early to bed, early to rise, have energy during day

   C. Have trouble falling to sleep, like staying up late at night, should nap

   D. Sleep late, sleepy after lunch, sometimes stay up late, naps make groggy

14. What is your favorite type of meal?

   A. Red meat, potatoes, vegetables, not big on sweets

   B. Seafood and chicken, vegetables, pasta, likes sweets

   C. Meat, likes traditional breakfast foods anytime, soups and stews

   D. Likes hearty food, root vegetables, chicken and grains, dessert with meals

15. What is your favorite time of year?

   A. Early spring and early fall, cool weather that promotes activity

   B. Winter and cold weather, snow

   C. Warm and wet, late spring or summer

   D. Cool fall, harvest time, early winter

16. Which of your five senses seems to be most active?

   A. Sight

   B. Touch

   C. Sound

   D. Smell/taste

17. What is your decision-making process?

    A. Quick decisions, go with gut, intuitive

    B. Take time to gather opinions, makes an emotional decision

    C. Snap assessments and decisions, but as new information is gathered may change mind

    D. Take time, think long and hard, once a decision is made may be stubborn about changing decision even with new information

18. What is your view of friendship?

    A. I make friends easily.

    B. My friendships are based on emotional connections.

    C. I have a lot of acquaintances but few friends.

    D. I'm cautious in friendship, but once a friend, always a friend.

19. Which of the following best describes your approach to rules of society?

    A. Rules are made to be broken or ignored.

    B. Rules should be followed but may need getting around on occasion.

    C. I will whine about the rules and encourage others to break them, but will follow them anyway.

    D. There must be a reason for the rules, so I'll follow them as they provide structure and safety until it is no longer safe.

20. Which of the following best describes your attitude toward money?

    A. I can always make more money, so I'll spend what I have.

    B. I'm going to be careful with my money to take care of my family.

    C. Money? I don't care about money. Maybe someone will give me some or I'll win the lottery.

    D. I spend frugally and save money for a rainy day.

You are all finished!

Add up all the As, Bs, Cs, and Ds to determine your elemental mix.

A=Fire

B=Water

C=Air

D=Earth

The letter with the most numbers is your dominant element and so on.

❧ AFTERWORD ❧

We are all born with seven talents. You've got to use all seven of your talents.

—Phyllis Light

LIKE KIDS WAITING for Santa Claus with baited breath, quite a few of us herbalists have been waiting for years for Phyllis Light to publish her work on southern folk medicine. Phyllis is one of the outstanding herbalists of our time. But she is not just a great practitioner and fount of wisdom. I'll tell you a secret: she's an "herb whisperer." The herbs live inside some people. When these people meet a little plant along the road a conversation might break out. It might not be in audible words: more like pictures, associations, and memories of cases, people, and constitutions—and suddenly, a new insight breaks out. Or it might just be, "Howdy down there!" "Thank you, how you all doing up there?" "Fine, thank you." The explosion of knowledge might come on another day. You never know.

One day Phyllis and I were walking through the woods in a park in her hometown. The ground slanted slightly to the north, so the woods were more like what I was familiar with in the Midwest, while the southern slopes were clad in the vegetation of the Deep South. "A perfect place to be an herbalist," I thought to myself. "You can pick in both regions only yards apart." As the reader will find out, Phyllis's herb knowledge reflects where she grew up—almost as if it sprang right up out of the ground.

We were looking at a wild yam vine tangled into the low-hanging branches of a white oak. The leaves come out in a whorl of six around the stem. Suddenly both of us had an insight. Many of the great Native American female medicines have three or six leaves, flower petals, or divisions in their terminal leaves—black cohosh, blue cohosh, trillium, raspberry, and wild yam. "How many pairs of tendons hold up the uterus?" I asked Phyllis.

The American Indian female medicines are one of the great "heritage gifts" of North American herbalism. In Europe, China, and India, there are four or five great female medicines in each tradition (lady's mantle, peony, cooked rehmannia root, shatavari) but in ours there are a dozen, learned in better times, when Native American healers and midwives taught their white and black neighbors about medicine plants—before the Trail of Tears and the terrible removals to the West. Before people forgot, or didn't care, or ignored the fact that Native people had an extra-sensory knowledge of wood and plant lore.

Phyllis is not just an herbalist, she is a conservator of the tradition in which she grew up—southern folk medicine. This heritage gift could easily be swept under the rug. Northerners think "Southern culture" is just an excuse for racism or backward-ism. They think theirs is the only legitimate culture and the "slow learners" will catch up one day. What they don't realize is that Southern culture is deep, different, and a little mysterious. In the North the "experts" are scientists and people with good diction, reflecting good education. In the South, Granny is an expert, and you better listen to your mama, 'cause what that scientist says may or may not be true. Anyway, Northerners don't really trust people that speak with a Southern accent, whether they be black or white—it's a dialect that sounds "rebellious" and "dangerous."

But Granny was right. She didn't put people on opioids, did she? Who's the danger here? The commercial/regulatory out-of-control monster system pampered by what I call "Northern folk culture"—or Granny? Can a monopoly see through the haze of its drug-infused, money-infected vision enough to judge Granny? No, it can't. Monopolies don't self-examine; their eyes look to the bottom line like magnets drawn to iron. Meanwhile, little herbs sneaking along the ground, like convicts on the run from pesticides and scientific facts, have more truth in their little green leaves than a system that can't come to terms with its financial addictions, can't listen to the people it is supposed to serve, can't tolerate what the patient says if it doesn't fit a defined category, can't acknowledge other forms of healing, can't understand the human condition except through lab tests and not imagination, art, emotion, intuition, instinct, or even sensation.

Phyllis Light is a *conscious* conservator of her culture and her healing heritage. She has studied her tradition in depth, bringing it into clarity in a time period when it could instead have lapsed into a final oblivion. And in giving her beloved tradition a voice she has done even more than that: she has given us a personal glimpse into what it was like to grow up in the Old South—not the South of gracious plantations, but of hardscrabble sharecropping, life-saving prayers, Holy Rollers, rattlesnake lore, and "sang hunting." She tells us why one "picks herbs" but "hunts ginseng."

I'm afraid that we herbalists will have to share our wonderful colleague and friend with a wider audience because—we could have predicted it—Phyllis has written a book that is fascinating beyond the little universe of the practicing herbalist.

—Matthew Wood
Martell, Wisconsin
"Up North"

❦ INDEX ❦

A

ADD/ADHD, 232
Adrenaline, 221, 226
African-Americans
    enslavement of, 82–85, 91
    Great Migration of, 94–95
    influence of, on Southern Folk
        Medicine, 82–85
Air
    breathing, 216–18
    characteristics of, 126
    deficient, 233–34
    excess, 231–33
    nature of, 222–24
    nervous system and, 218–20
    neurotransmitters and, 225–27
    traits, 228–30
    wind vs., 214–16, 219, 222
Akenson, Donald Harman, 85
Alabama tribe, 80
Aldosterone, 206, 207
Allostasis, 28
Almanac Man. *See* The Signs
Aloe vera, 4, 106
Alternative medicine, definition of, 11
American Medical Association, 10
Anger, 183
Anise, 106
Antidotes, 129–30
Antioxidants, 173, 179
Apprenticeships, 18–19

Asclepius, Cult of, 69–70
Astrology
    constitutional makeup and, 161
    folk, 107–10
ATP (adenosine triphosphate), 31, 172, 174,
    216-18, 217, 244
Audubon, John James, 153
Avavares, 102–3
Avicenna, 60, 71
Ayurveda, 13, 72

B

Bacon, Francis, 135
Bass, Arthur Lee "Tommie"
    herbal practice of, 22–25
    illness classification and, 37
    life of, 21–22
    parents of, 89
    personality of, 21, 24–25
    quotations of, 1, 21, 25, 34
    recognition of, 23
    training of, 22
Bass's Salve, 23–24
Bay laurel, 106–7
Beecher, Donald, 66
Berly, William, 91
Bernard, Claude, 26–27, 30
The Bible
    as healing tool, 104–5
    herbs in, 105–7

✾ ABOUT THE AUTHOR ✾

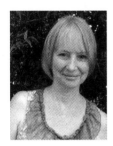 PHYLLIS D. LIGHT, MA, RH (AHG), is a fourth-generation herbalist and healer. Her studies in Southern and Appalachian folk medicine began at the age of ten in the deep woods of North Alabama with lessons from her Creek/Cherokee grandmother, and continued with well-known folk herbalist Tommie Bass. She received a master of health studies from the University of Alabama. Light is a registered herbalist and currently acts as vice president of the American Herbalist Guild and as a member of the admissions committee. She is also the president of the American Naturopathic Certification Board. Locally, Light is the director of the Appalachian Center for Natural Health in Arab, Alabama, which offers both online and residential classes.

Learn more at phyllisdlight.com.

About North Atlantic Books

North Atlantic Books (NAB) is an independent, nonprofit publisher committed to a bold exploration of the relationships between mind, body, spirit, and nature. Founded in 1974, NAB aims to nurture a holistic view of the arts, sciences, humanities, and healing. To make a donation or to learn more about our books, authors, events, and newsletter, please visit www.northatlanticbooks.com.

North Atlantic Books is the publishing arm of the Society for the Study of Native Arts and Sciences, a 501(c)(3) nonprofit educational organization that promotes cross-cultural perspectives linking scientific, social, and artistic fields. To learn how you can support us, please visit our website.